The Art and Practice
of Low Vision

The Art and Practice of Low Vision

by
Paul B. Freeman, O.D. F.A.A.O.
Diplomate Low Vision

Randall T. Jose, O.D. F.A.A.O.
Diplomate Low Vision

with special contributions by
Greg Goodrich, Ph.D., F.A.A.O.

Butterworth–Heinemann
Boston   London   Oxford   Singapore   Sydney   Toronto   Wellington

Library of Congress Cataloging-in-Publication Data

Freeman, Paul B.
The art and practice of low vision/ by Paul B. Freeman, Randall T. Jose,
with special contributions by Greg Goodrich.
        p.   cm.
Includes bibliographical references and index.
ISBN 0–7506–9010–0 (pbk. : acid-free paper)
    1. Low vision—Patients—Rehabilitation.   2. Optometry.   I. Jose, Randall T., 1943–   .
II. Goodrich, Greg.   III. Title.
RE91.FG7   1991
617.7—dc20

                                                    90–25599
                                                    CIP

British Library Cataloguing in Publication Data

Freeman, Paul B.
    The art and practice of low vision.
    I. Opthalmology
    I. Title   II. Jose, Randall T.   III. Goodrich, Greg
    617.7

    ISBN 0–7506–9010–0

Butterworth–Heinemann
80 Montvale Avenue
Stoneham, MA 02180

Printed in the United States of America

Contents

Foreword

This is a book for the general practitioner who includes low-vision patients in his practice, but hasn't discovered the secret of being happy doing this work. This book is also for practitioners who may have considered doing low-vision work, but have no idea how to start up or organize such a practice.

The emphasis in these pages is on organizing an office to cope with the problems and feelings of low-vision patients, and on incorporating the care of low-vision patients into a general practice structure. If we understand the psychological problems of a person with impaired vision, we can create an atmosphere in the office that is reassuring. If we direct the examination, instruction, and prescription toward helping the patient adjust, we are fulfilling our goal of vision rehabilitation.

Whether the practitioner is an old-hand or a newcomer to low vision, there are many practical suggestions for everyone in these chapters. I have found the use of model letters to patients, and the use of referral sources, community resources, and checklists to be invaluable. Letters can be used to introduce patients to low-vision procedures, and to start patients out with a much more realistic attitude toward the low-vision experience. Other letters can be used to thank people for referrals. If you are very busy, you may neglect to dictate a thanks-for-referral letter for a couple of weeks. With a nice-looking model letter, the details can be filled in quickly, and the thank you letter can be on the way in the next mail.

This book does not try to do any more than outline the ingredients of the exam, the essential function tests, and the equipment and devices needed. Technique is suggested, but choices are still up to the individual practitioner and style of practice.

The wide selection of training sheets for homework and home training are valuable if there are patients in the practice who need this type of reinforcement.

The emphasis is very much on the patient, as it should be. The patient, by participating in filling out pre-examination and history forms, starts with a reality base which saves the practitioner a lot of unnecessary backtracking to undo unrealistic expectations. When reviewing this material I was reminded of how easy it is to forget how lost a patient feels, how frustrated, and how long it takes to adjust. The average clinician cannot and should not spend lengthy sessions with a patient. Neither can an instructor be expected to pick up clues immediately. But if the patient has time to review and think over the material provided for her in advance, the therapeutic process can take place where it should—in the patient's own mind, with support from those persons close to the patient. Working with family or friends introduces another type of reinforcement for the patient— that of a family relationship or a shared activity with a friend.

Rehabilitation of any type does not necessarily lead to happy patients, but the well-informed person who participates fully in his therapy learns to accept and work with his limitations with a better understanding.

The *Art and Practice of Low Vision* is what its title says it is. It does not attempt to introduce yet another method of doing low vision, but rather tries to fill in the important spaces that are generally glossed over in texts on low vision; that is, how to make it fit into a busy practice and be successful and satisfying.

Eleanor E. Faye, MD FACS

Preface

The Art and Practice of Low Vision is a how-to book oriented for the clinician who wants either to begin or enhance a low-vision practice.

This book is organized in a way that the practitioner is walked through the steps of a low-vision practice. We provide forms and hand-outs that should not only make the clinician's venture into a low-vision practice easier but should also provide patients with optimum care. The concepts presented are based on our clinical experience. For those readers who wish to understand the more academic aspects of the clinical information presented, we direct your attention to the Appendix which contains additional bibliographic resources and materials.

Usually the primary goal of a low-vision patient who seeks help is to be able to read again. The ability to read print is an important part of an individual's effort to maintain an independent life. Yet many low-vision patients who look for help misunderstand the nature of the help they can get from optical devices and quickly become discouraged. They confuse the ability to recognize letters with the ability to read in a normal way.

It is a thrilling moment when a person who is visually impaired can sit in an examination chair, look through a pair of lenses, and actually see letters again. But of course, reading requires much more—speed, fluency, comprehension—and it may take months of practice to attain these. It also takes recognition of what the reading goals are; they may differ from person to person. One patient may want to be able to read the directions for knitting a sweater without having to ask someone for help, while another may want to read several mystery novels a week. Their actual vision may be identical, but it may take considerably more effort on the part of the latter patient to achieve that desired goal.

Although the primary goal of a low-vision patient is reading, many also want to view objects in the distance, i.e., bus signs, TV, fast-food wall menus, or friends' faces. It is exciting for a visually impaired person to see 20/20, but seeing a stationary chart and becoming visually functional are worlds apart.

The goal of the low-vision practitioner is to help low-vision patients understand the nature of the rehabilitative process and to help them meet their individual goals whenever possible. This is done by providing careful evaluations of the impairment, making relevant recommendations for low-vision devices, giving exercises that will assist patient progress, and tracking this progress through follow-up examinations.

We hope this book will serve as a starting point for many low-vision or potential low-vision practitioners. Once the reader acquires more experience and more patient contact, the information from this book (along with other books in the field) will help to further enhance patient care.

Acknowledgments

A book of this nature could not have been written without the help either directly or indirectly of several people. We would like to express our appreciation to Dee Quillman, John Ferraro, and Leslie Piqueras for their considerable impact on this work. In the field of low vision any truly great work is done through a multidisciplinary team effort. These individuals help exemplify that concept.

We would also like to thank all those who have written in the field of low vision. Without those erudite individuals, works like this could not have been envisioned. We would especially like to thank, as a group, the low-vision diplomates of the American Academy of Optometry. It is through interacting with this merry band of concerned practitioners that we were able to bounce many of our ideas around.

This type of work cannot be done without the labor of readers, typists, and all-around helpers. Thanks to Michelle Gernat and Pat Miller for the hours spent helping to do the tough job of reading, rereading, and typing.

Finally, we would like to thank our wives, Barbara and Maryann, who have helped us redefine the quality of life.

Introduction

Before you begin to examine a low-vision patient, there is certain terminology, equipment, and managerial information you should be familiar with.

Definition of Services

To start with you must first define for yourself, and later to your patients, what the service you are performing is and what a low-vision examination is not. Following is a definition for consideration when explaining to your patient what you do, why it is different, and why a team approach is necessary.

What a Low-Vision Evaluation Is   A low-vision evaluation is a functional evaluation to determine whether the vision that you presently have can be improved to do those activities that you wish to do. This evaluation will include an exploration of both optical and nonoptical systems available to assist in maximizing your vision.

What a Low-Vision Evaluation Is Not   A low-vision evaluation is not a medical evaluation to determine eye health. This evaluation should have been done by your referring practitioner as the justification for additional specialized services. It is imperative that you have a primary-care optometrist or ophthalmologist who is, has, and will monitor your eyes for any eye conditions which could result in additional eye health complications or additional vision loss. You must continue to be evaluated by your referring doctor over regular intervals of time.

Scheduling

Scheduling a low-vision patient can be tricky. The reason is because the patient's first visit must incorporate a number of areas of concern—what the patient wants, your basic findings, a summarization of what you have done, a discussion of the direction you wish to pursue with the patient, etc. Typically, initial evaluations should be allotted an hour to an hour and a half. Even if the time allotted is greater than the time needed, the remaining time can be used to discuss any concerns the patient might have about the condition creating low vision, practitioner referral information, family interactive information, etc.

Subsequent Scheduling

Subsequent scheduling should be done to include tests that were not done on the first visit, any verification procedures that you wish to perform, and/or vision therapy and stimulation activities that the patient may need. This session typically should be scheduled for 30 to 45 minutes. Remember during each visit the patient may give you information which could require modification in the management plan and ultimate prescription for the patient. Allow for these modifications.

Additionally, there are some tests that need to be done at every visit from both a legal and measurement perspective, i.e., visual acuities, intraocular pressure, and any other test that you feel will be necessary to maintain a perspective on the patient's eye health and progress.

Equipment Needs

Typically, the primary goal of most patients is reading or other near activities. As a result, near lenses need to be available for the patient as well as telescopes for distance evaluation. The following is a list of low-vision devices that one might want to obtain. It is important to realize that one should be proficient in prescribing low-vision devices before building a large stock of systems. An initial outlay can be as much or as little as you wish.

Equipment

Several companies offer kits to initiate the practitioner to the practice of low vision (Designs for Vision, Coburn Optical Industries, Duffens, F/V Microscopes, Eschenbach). Most of the kits are geared toward the company's products. The practitioner will need diagnostic equipment in each of the following treatment option areas.

1. full-field microscopes 2x to 12x
2. prismatic half-eyes +4 to +12
3. hand-held magnifiers 2x to 5x
4. pocket magnifiers 4x to 10x
5. stand magnifiers 3x to 8x
6. illuminated stand magnifiers 6x to 12x
7. halogen-illuminated magnifiers 6x to 12x
8. hand-held telescopes 2.5x to 10x
9. spectacle mounted telescopes 2.0x to 6.0x
10. binocular spectacle telescopes 3.0x
11. near binocular telemicroscopes 3x, 4x
12. bioptics 3x to 6x
13. binoculars (monocular) 7x to 18x
14. filters
15. closed-circuit television (CCTV)
16. special diagnostic charts, contrast sensitivity chart, etc.
17. loaners

These kits can range from a modest $1000 to meet an occasional primary-care need to $20,000 for a comprehensive set to meet all needs (including loaners).

Loaner System

A loaner system is a must. Patients who perform well in the office will not always perform equally as well at home. Regardless of how much training is done in the office, there are environmental considerations that the doctor cannot be made aware of unless the patient is allowed to take the devices home. Obviously there are some systems like a closed-circuit television or some of the more sophisticated telescopes that cannot be readily loaned out.

The loaner system takes the burden of "forced success" away from both the practitioner and the patient. As long as the system is loaned, neither member of the doctor-patient team will feel the pressure of creating perceived success. After using a loaner system, it's prescription and purchase will have been done with the knowledge of its advantages and limitations both in and out of the office. If on the other hand the patient is prescribed a system prior to a trial with a loaner, the doctor might feel the need to continue to "push" the device in an effort to avoid refunding the patient's money. Or the patient may feel the doctor has simply sold a device to the patient without proper trial.

Staff

Initially a low-vision practitioner should do every activity that is involved in the low-vision evaluation from intake, to evaluation, to training. Once the practitioner is fully comfortable with the total process, then other staff members can be called on to perform parts in the evaluation. Using sophisticated staff, i.e., orientation and mobility specialists, social workers, occupational therapists, and physical therapists, is wonderful but not always practical. However, these services should be available to you and your patients in your community.

Fee Structure

The fee structure in low-vision treatment should be similar in concept to any other part of an individual's practice. All aspects of what is involved in an examination should be considered before arriving at a fee. The patient should be thoroughly informed about these fees at the time of the initial contact, which is usually by phone.

Patients should also be made aware of third-party reimbursement. Optometrists have entered into the third-party reimbursement arena. By doing that, optometrists must understand that third-party carriers follow certain guidelines regardless of the speciality of the doctor. Following are some guidelines to help the optometrist through the third-party payor maze:

1. Third-party carriers do not typically cover those services that revolve around routine evaluations. Coverage is designed to assist those that are in need of care due to a medically necessary condition. The low-vision patient typically, by definition, is one who has a decreased visual acuity or reduced visual field due to a medically diagnosed condition of the visual system and should fit into most profiles that third-party carriers have regarding medical necessity. It is incumbent upon the optometrist, however, to understand the language the third-party carriers use to reimburse either the practitioner or the patient.

2. Low vision, in almost all instances, is not a covered service. The reason is that low vision is not a disease. It is the end result of a disease. It is advisable, therefore, not to use low vision as a diagnosis or type of service. Do not try to convince the carrier to cover this speciality or the phrase *low vision*.

3. Most carriers need one diagnosis to reimburse a patient or doctor for the service. Listing more than one diagnosis will not impress the person who enters the information into the computer, and in fact, could lead to reasons why certain tests might not be covered based on confusion due to a specific pathology(s) as it relates to services rendered.

4. The doctor who is planning to submit for a specific service should first find out whether that service is covered in the locality that the practitioner is practicing. This can usually be found out by contacting the carrier directly. Consultative visits, office visits, and the level of those visits are not necessarily covered by all carriers in all sections of the country. Rather than frustrating and/or embarrassing both practitioner and patient, it is advisable to be clear on what services are covered.

5. For those services that are consultative in nature, it is important to review item 4 above. In addition, a consultation typically applies to the first visit. Any visit following a consultation, according to most carriers, is considered an office visit—the level depends upon the type of service being rendered. In addition, there are certain requirements that a consultation has that other visits do not. Some of these are

   • The practitioner must render advice to the patient.
   • The practitioner must write a report.
   • The practitioner may not prescribe at a consultation visit unless the referring doctor has requested that it be done.

6. Any special services that a doctor wishes to perform and wants covered by third-party carriers must be justified not only in the mind of the practitioner but, equally as importantly, in the mind of the carrier. As an example, taking a picture of the fundus of a cataract patient, when cataract is the diagnosis being used, may not be covered because of the lack of relationship between a

fundus photo and cataract in the mind of the third-party carrier. In the final analysis, anything can be rejected by the third-party carrier and then must be justified by the practitioner.

7. Being creative is not always good. Using codes that are not optometric or ophthalmological, even if they work, can lead to trouble. Third-party carriers who have made mistakes can come back at a later date to collect those funds (and possible interest) even if they find they are in error.

8. Using maximum reimbursable codes over multiple visits will send up a red flag and will either cause the carrier to deny payment or will invite a visit from a third-party payor for an explanation of services. An example of this is overutilizing comprehensive office visits. This assumes you have provided every available service for each of those visits.

9. Presently, low-vision devices are not reimbursable. However, some practitioners have tried and been successful in receiving reimbursement by writing a narrative along with a diagnosis. But, don't be surprised if the majority of the time the claim is denied.

These guidelines will be useful in helping the low-vision practitioner legitimately maximize and justify the use of third-party payors for the benefit of the patient as well as the practitioner.

1 | Before the Initial Examination

The phone rings, and a low-vision patient or family member makes an appointment or a referring doctor's office schedules one of their patients for your services. Once the appointment has been made, communication becomes an integral part of your initial contact with the patient. Before you actually examine the patient, several pieces of correspondence should be written. In this section, we examine the order and the kind of letters you will be writing. On the following pages are examples of letters you can use to communicate with your patient, the referring doctor or other referral source, and the patient's spouse or helper. You can also design your own forms using these as guides.

CONTENTS

FORM DESCRIPTIONS

1.1 Thank You for Your Referral
The first letter you will need to write is to the referring doctor or other referral source. Not only is this good public relations, but it also lets the referring source know the appointment has been made.

1.2 Thank You for Your Help
At the time the appointment is made, find out if there is a person who can help the patient read materials you will be sending before the initial examination. The Thank You for Your Help letter should accompany the appointment form so that the patient's spouse, relative, or friend can help with the information sent.

1.3 History Form
Additional materials that can be enclosed with the Thank You for Your Help letter include a map and an initial Brief History form to be filled out.

The history is a method of obtaining introductory background information necessary to help you understand the patient better and decide what procedural modifications you might have to make to achieve your patient's goals. This history can be sent with the appointment information. Many clinicians have a high compliance rate from patients who fill out the history form prior to the evaluation. Remember that a more formal history will be taken in the office with the patient.

1.4 About Your Appointment

Along with this material, you should include the information contained in the patient handout About Your Appointment. This handout includes instructions about what the patient should bring to the initial examination as well as provides information on setting realistic treatment goals. If you have the capability, sending these patient materials in large-print format (i.e., 14-point typeface) may help patients respond independently to the questions asked, assuring them even before the evaluation that you have thought about potential methods of visual assistance. This is a great boost to establishing good doctor-patient rapport.

THANK YOU FOR YOUR REFERRAL

Thank you for referring _____ for a low-vision evaluation. I appreciate the confidence you have in my services and will endeavor to continue to practice at the highest level of eye care for the visually impaired. _____ is scheduled to be seen on _____ 19____. I will keep you informed of our services as they are provided. Again, thank you for referring _____ and allowing me the opportunity to share in your patient's vision care.

Sincerely,

1.2

THANK YOU FOR YOUR HELP

Dear

This information has been sent to help _____ prepare for
a low-vision evaluation. Reading this may be difficult, if not impossible for
_____. I would appreciate it, and I'm sure _____ would appreciate
your help in reading this to (him/her.) As you read this you will begin to get a
sense of the potential help for _____ and what will be involved.

Thank you in advance for your assistance.

Sincerely,

BRIEF HISTORY

Can you read print?	Yes	No
Can you watch television?	Yes	No
Can you travel independently?	Yes	No
Are you taking medicine?	Yes	No

List

_____

_____

_____

_____

_____

Does sunlight bother your eyes?   Yes   No

Additional comments:

ABOUT YOUR APPOINTMENT

Welcome

You have made an appointment for a low-vision examination. This will be one of the most important appointments you will make for improving your ability to see. So that you can get the most from the examination, I am sending you this handout which explains how you can assist me and my staff to best serve you.

First, you must realize there are no miracles. Your lost vision cannot be restored. Low vision is a rehabilitation process. That means you are going to be taught how to effectively use your remaining vision.

You can be helped to use your remaining vision in three different ways.

1. Learn to use your remaining vision more efficiently than you do now. There are many eye movement skills that you will learn to help you do this.
2. Utilize alternative devices to perform certain tasks. These include better lighting, high contrast, enlarged print, and auditory or hearing techniques.
3. Use special optical lenses such as magnifiers, spectacle microscopes, and telescopes. These will improve your ability to see detail (read or watch TV) but may require you to hold material close to your eyes or see through only a small field of view. However, the benefits usually far outweigh the limitations if you really want to see.

Preparing for the Appointment

It will be helpful to me if you think about specific problems you are having at home, work, or school because of your failing vision. This may include problems with reading, watching TV, getting around, playing cards, sewing, knitting, woodworking, or other social and recreational activities. Some of these problems may not be helped by the options available, but we won't know if you don't tell us. Think about those things that you would like to see better. Start to think in terms of goals. It will be helpful to *write down problem areas* or have the person reading this write them down for you along with the goals you hope to attain.

The examination may be lengthy. Ask the receptionist approximately how long your visit will take so that you can plan for this extended visit. Make sure you schedule around your medications and meals, and select a time when you feel your vision is at it's best.

What to Bring to the Examination

Bring any glasses or magnifying glasses you are presently using. If you have any special materials (forms, books, needlepoint, etc.) you want to be able to work with, bring them to the examination as well. This is particularly important for materials you use at work, school, or for those hobbies that you might wish to pursue.

Finally

This will be your initial visit. I will need to see you several times to make sure that you are getting the best prescription for your eyes and that the goals you want to accomplish are attained. It also gives me time to loan you a device to use at home prior to prescribing the final one. This added home experience will allow us to design the low-vision device that will provide you with the best performance and greatest comfort.

Keep in mind through this experience that the best low-vision service occurs when you form a partnership with me, one where both of us understand your goals and work together to attain them.

2 | The Initial Low-Vision Examination and Evaluation

This chapter will help you organize a low-vision examination. It outlines the initial or consultation visit in two parts. The first part covers all the tests and forms you will need to conduct the initial examination. The second part shows how this information should be used to form a low-vision device evaluation. Both discussions are in the form of a clinical introduction, as there are excellent books in the literature that cover the more extensive and theoretical issues related to the examination (see the Appendix for listing).

CONTENTS

INITIAL EXAMINATION

All low-vision practitioners have their own methods of evaluating low-vision patients. The following guideline for the low-vision evaluation is exactly that—a guideline. There are many factors that have specifically not been considered in this discussion. You will have to modify and improvise based on your patient's age, both chronological and developmental, and on any additional impairments and the communication abilities of your patient. Hopefully, as you develop your practice and establish a philosophy of care for the visually impaired individual, you will modify this guide and redesign it to fit your approach.

Before you begin the examination you will also want to be sure you've received a filled-out copy of the patient's Brief History Form (form 1.3), which the patient should have received in the information packet before the initial visit. Use this information along with the cover sheet (form 2.1) to establish a well-organized patient file. A formal history should also be taken when the patient is in the office (form 2.2). Included in this form is an example of typical questions to be asked during the consultation. Initially they can be used verbatim. As you gain experience, you can develop personal phrases to elicit the information. Every item should be explored until you are satisfied that you have enough information to formulate a plan of treatment for your patient. The patient's primary and secondary goals are those parts of the history that will direct your evaluation.

The initial consultation is diagnostic in nature. With the information from the history and examination forms in hand, you will have a feel for the handicapping effect of the patient's visual loss. Your job, as a low-vision clinician, is to minimize this handicap. To do that, you must know and understand the extent and impact of the impairment (loss) so that you can describe your patient's visual functioning. The examination procedures described in this chapter will give you that information. You will demonstrate your expertise and encourage the patient's confidence in your abilities. Throughout the examination, you should be thinking about magnification, field of view, lighting needs, working distance, contrast needs, and skills necessary to accomplish the goals of your patient.

EXAMINATION PROCEDURES

Distance Visual Acuity Testing

As in any other type of eye examination, acuity testing should be done monocularly and binocularly. Typically, this is done with the old prescription and/or without any prescription. You will note that lighting conditions should be reported. They will be important in your closing remarks when discussing environment.

Testing distances (2 $\frac{1}{2}$, 5, 10 feet, etc.) for visual acuities are individual, but success-oriented acuities are necessary to maintain a positive approach to the evaluation. Typically, testing is performed at 10 feet, unless the acuities are below 20/400; then closer distances of 5 or 2 to 2 $\frac{1}{2}$ feet will provide better results. The acuity test is an important psychological as well as physiological test, so make sure the patient is able to read numbers or letters on the chart instead of counting fingers. *Counting fingers is a negative way to obtain an acuity.* A patient who can see your fingers can respond to a chart acuity at the same distance. Encourage guessing and tell the patient to "move the eye around" to see the figures on the chart better. If you can improve the acuity a line or two by exposing only one line at a time, the patient will most likely benefit from eccentric viewing training.

There are many types of acuity charts used to test low vision. If acuities other than Snellen are done, they should be noted in parentheses after the acuity, i.e., (Feinbloom visual acuities). This signifies that the testing was done using Feinbloom visual acuity charts.

Some excellent clinical charts for low-vision patients are the Feinbloom Distant Number Chart; Bailey-Lovie Chart; Bailey Hi-Low Contrast Chart; Lighthouse Symbol Cards; and Efron Symbol Cards. Most of these are available through the New York Lighthouse Low Vision Products or Multi-Media Center at the School of Optometry, University of California at Berkeley.

Remember, for legal purposes acuities should be converted to Snellen equivalents. Record the actual measurement and the equi-valent acuity in parentheses, i.e., 10/60 (20/120). These acuities are valuable for teachers, rehabilitation specialists, etc.

Off-Center Acuities

Distance acuity measurement varies not only by distance but by position of view. If someone has a central or multiple scotomas, then eccentric viewing techniques are necessary. Watch for patients trying to find that best spot on their own, and note that. However, you may have to guide the patient. It may be useful to start a line or two above your estimate of the patient's visual acuity so that the patient has some practice on easier lines before getting to threshold. The authors have found some alterna-tives to having the patient view "around the blind spot."

One is to hold the chart directly in front of the patient. When the patient attempts to see the numbers, letters, or object on the chart, quickly move the chart laterally. This puts the chart information in an eccentric position rather than having the patient move his eye to that position.

Another alternative is to hold your hand above the line on the chart you want the patient to read. Instruct the patient to look at your hand, and while doing so, read the numbers on the chart below. Typically, the superior position will elicit a good response and will be a good demon-stration of eccentric viewing for a patient who has not learned this tech-nique yet. The clinician can also evaluate fixation to the left and inferior. Avoid viewing to the right of fixation.

Starting Optics

This information, i.e., visual acuities at distance, should help you to think about calculating not only a distance but a near starting point for optical consideration. At distance if a patient has 20/200 and needs to see 20/50, then a 4x telescopic arrangement will be necessary ($200 \div 50 = 4$). If you decide that the patient needs to see 20/40 at near, then using the Brazelton formula will give you a starting point for near magnifiers; i.e., 20/200 distance, and you want 20/40 at near. Take the denominator of the distance and divide it by the denominator of what you want for near. You will arrive at a magnification of 5x ($200 \div 40 = 5x$).

Contrast Sensitivity Function (CSF) Testing

Two patients with the same Snellen acuity can function differently. This difference can usually be predicted with contrast sensitivity testing. In general, a poor contrast indicates that the clinician should give more attention to glare control, contrast of viewing materials, and illumination. These factors are often more important than magnification. A patient can be doing poorly with a 3x magnifier, but by adding a halogen light to the 3x, optimum visual functioning can be achieved. Without the light, it might take 5x magnification to achieve the same acuity performance. Do not deny your patient optimum visual performance by neglecting CSF tests.

The Vistech charts, as an example, are most valuable when the patient is tested at 1 meter. A patient with 20/200 and a normal CSF curve will respond better than a patient with 20/160 and an abnormal curve. Loss of high-frequency contrast usually indicates problems with near point and reading tasks. More light is needed, and specially designed lenses (doublet, Volk) with less light loss are optimum. Telemicroscopes are very poor choices as a prescription in these cases. Low-frequency losses usually indicate problems with mobility and travel-related tasks. The Bailey Hi-Low Contrast Acuity Chart or the Peli Robson Chart are other easy ways to screen for the presence of a contrast problem. Reading only the first two lines on the Peli Robson chart or dropping more than two lines of acuity from the 100% contrast to the 10% contrast on the Bailey Hi-Lo Chart indicates that there is a significant problem with contrast. These two tests are not as diagnostic as the Vistech test, but very practical to administer in terms of cost and time. Issues of lighting, filters, and optimum full-field optical-systems need to be considered in designing the prescription. Contrast sensitivity is an important measurement of vision that should not be overlooked by the low-vision clinician.

Near Acuity Testing

Because the majority of your clinical population is interested in near activities, specifically reading, it is incumbent upon you to measure near acuities. There are numerous charts available with single letters, multiple letters, numbers, words, phrases, sentences, etc. A good starting point is to use a chart with single numbers or letters. This will provide the best acuity and be psychologically reinforcing for the patient. You can then do near acuities both with and without a typoscope. A typoscope is a black card with a window cut out of it, large enough to view a line of letters, words, etc. (available at Designs for Vision, New York Lighthouse Low Vision Products, etc.). If using the typoscope allows the patient to show a significant improvement in acuity (paragraph charts especially), you should consider contrast-enhancing devices and/or eccentric viewing training prior to evaluating magnification. Remember that the distance from the near chart must be noted. Watch for the need to view eccentrically. Lighting is a consideration and should be identified for later use in discussions of the environment.

The best near acuity chart to start with is the Lighthouse Near Acuity Chart. It was designed to be used at 40 cm. If one holds the chart at 40 cm, it is easy to convert acuities into magnification by using the diopters listed on the right-hand side of the chart. The Snellen acuities on this chart were calculated on a 40-cm working distance as indicated by the instructional data written on the chart. Therefore if one uses that distance, magnification is represented by the formula $M = D/2.5$, or every 2.5D equals 1 times magnification.

Think about calculating a near starting lens using this information. It is fairly straightforward. Take your measurement at a specific distance (40 cm for this example). Record in M notation, i.e., 5M at 40 cm. Using the 40 cm or +2.5 diopters reference, multiply 2.5 x 5M for a starting magnification of +12.5D. If you want to be lazy, simply read the 12D notation on the right-hand side of the chart. If, however, you choose to use a different initial measurement distance, then you must modify the diopter multiplier for the new reference distance.*

The chart below shows examples using 40, 33, or 25 cm as test distances.

Using a different example one can see how a different distance will affect magnification. A patient reading 3M at 33 cm with best correction will need an initial add of +9 diopters. Put this in a trial frame; hold the chart at 11 cm, and the patient should read 1M letters.

Another method of determining an initial level of magnification is to have the patient read the chart at a comfortable distance. Record the M

	Test distance:	40 cm	33 cm	25 cm
	Magnification:	D/2.5	D/3	D/4
Patient's Acuity	1M	2.50D	3D	4D
	2M	5.00D	6D	8D
	3M	7.50D	9D	12D
	4M	10.00D	12D	16D
	5M	12.50D	15D	20D
	6M	15.00D	18D	24D
	etc	**Diopter Add required to read 1M print**		

*D/4 was originally used because 25 cm was considered to be a standard work distance. To see at 25 cm one would need to exert 4D of accommodation or use a +4.00D add or a combination of accommodation and lens power to achieve the unit of magnification 1, i.e., $M = D/4$, $M = 4/4$ or 1. Obviously if one needed more magnification one would need to move in closer therefore requiring more accommodation and lens power. However, because not everyone uses 25 cm as the distance from which to start, the denominator of the magnification formula will change with the working distance.

print size and test distance. Suppose the patient reads 5M at 30 cm and you want 1M to be read. This requires 5x magnification. This can be achieved by moving the print 5x closer. At 6 cm (30/5 = 6 cm) the patient must accommodate approximately 16D (100/6 = 16.6D). Therefore, you should start your evaluation using a +16D lens at 6 cm. (This happens to be equivalent to a 4x microscope using the standard D/4 formula used by manufacturers, but the clinician will stay out of trouble if all work is done in diopters.) If the patient reads 1M at 6 cm, this is a potential prescription, and training can be initiated. If 1.5M is read, the clinician should check the work distance, uncorrected cylinder, lighting, contrast, eccentric viewing problems, metamorphopsia, etc. There should be some reason the patient cannot achieve this theoretical result. Try evaluating these other factors before increasing magnification. If the patient holds the material at 4 cm instead of 6 cm and the material is in focus, the clinician should consider the need for more magnification (the patient is accommodating) or consider the possibility that the patient is an uncorrected myope (recheck the distant refraction). A consistent 8 cm work distance may also indicate uncorrected hyperopia. As you can see, there is more to acuity testing than getting a number! Also remember that manufacturers' statements of magnification are often unreliable, so you may need to be flexible in selecting the magnifier that meets your calculated value; i.e., you may find that a 5x magnifier actually gives you 4x magnification.

Binocular Testing

The majority of visually impaired patients are monocular. You, however, need to assess ocular alignment to determine the possibility for developing or maintaining binocular vision (or simultaneous perception) where this can be achieved. Some patients are biocular; they can use either eye independently while suppressing the other. This is typical of an alternating strabismus. This condition may allow you to prescribe a telescope for one eye and a microscope for the other eye.

Even if your patient is monocular, with 20/60 in one eye and 20/600 in the other, it is often necessary to occlude the poorer eye to obtain maximum acuity, especially when using microscopes. Sometimes retinal rivalry exists, and unless the poorer eye is occluded, the patient will report, among other things, a blur, jumping print, or poor localization. Sometimes a patient may even need to close the poorer eye to reduce interference by physically closing it with a hand.

Binocularity or a simultaneous perception can exist if the acuities are within two lines of one another. A Cover test and a Hirschberg test will show motor alignment. Worth Four Dot testing will show gross fusion. If the patient shows even gross stereopsis (as a result of Stereo Fly testing), the clinician should make extra efforts to attain and/or sustain binocular vision. Summation of the CSF curve when tested binocularly is also a strong indication that the clinician should strive for a binocular prescription (Rx).

Color Vision Testing   This testing can be done in a multitude of ways, the simplest of which is matching or identifying yarn, as in the Holmgren test. While not scientific in nature, this testing will give functional information as to how the patient performs in his everyday environment. If you want to be more scientific, remember to monitor the type of light being used. A more diagnostic test is the Large Disc D-15 test (available from the Blind Rehabilitation Center in Birmingham or Dr. Paul Pease at the University of Houston College of Optometry). Most patients can respond to this test, and it provides excellent functional data related to color vision problems that may affect the patient's ability to perform vocational/educational tasks. It is administered and interpreted in basically the same manner as the regular D-15 test.

Field Testing

While the patient is sitting in the chair, both monocular and binocular confrontation fields should be performed at 1 meter. This is more functionally than pathologically oriented, giving you, the patient, and others in the room an understanding of the patient's field of view. Those who want to do more in-depth fields should do so by using any of the more sophisticated tests available. Remember, in the low-vision examination you are more interested in mobility or functional visual fields. More sophisticated field tests to determine the nature of a specific scotoma for following the pathology should have been done by the referring doctor, or will need to be done at a separate visit.

The evaluation of visual fields can provide you with information regarding the extent of intact central retina available for magnification. It does not do any good to magnify within scotomas. In addition, the visual fields will help explain why a patient might not have responded as well as expected to the telescopic or microscopic magnification. It will give you insight into the ability of an optical system to resolve identified problems. For instance, a 3° to 5° field may place limitations on the amount of magnification that can be useful to the patient. Patients with fields of 5° to 10° with good part-whole perceptual skills are good candidates for most magnification, as these fields put moderate limits on the patient's visual performance. (*Note*: Mobility training is typically needed by individuals with fields of 40° or less.) To function effectively with a low-vision device, some additional training may be needed for patients with small fields. Fields that are 10° or larger are usually no problem relative to the use of optical devices.

Perimetry should be evaluated in patients who show peripheral restrictions with confrontation testing. Large targets 6 to 20 mm round should be used as needed to get a response. An X made of tape across the point of fixation will help the patient with nystagmus or a central scotoma fixate a little more accurately. Extend the X as far as is necessary for the patient to view the lines and understand how to visualize where the X would cross if visible. Tell your patient with a central scotoma to look where the lines of the cross appear to intersect. Only eight or ten meridians need to be evaluated. Modifications that can be made to the programs of some of the newer automated field testers make it possible to perform even more sophisticated field studies without fatiguing the patient. Also the new threshold field studies provide excellent information pertaining to the quality of vision and eccentric viewing strategies but are usually too time-consuming to be incorporated in a primary-care low-vision practice.

Amsler Grid Testing

This test can be administered after the refraction. Some clinicians prefer to do this at the time of the near acuity evaluation. The testing should be done monocularly and binocularly using the appropriate lens for the viewing distance. The patient should hold the grid close enough to see the fixation dot. Record this distance. (If each square is 1° at 33 cm, then it will represent 3° at 11 cm). The patient is told to describe any areas of the chart where boxes are missing (indicating scotoma) or areas of the chart where the boxes are distorted (indicating metamorphopsia) while fixating on the central dot. Some clinicians use the chart with the large fixational cross to help patients locate the dot and hold fixation. Sometimes an Amsler grid on a light box will help obtain more reliable responses.

The goal of this procedure is to obtain functional rather than pathological information, i.e., eccentric viewing. The information from this test, i.e., indications of metamophopsia, blur, scotoma, will impact your ultimate low-vision prescription. Examples of this are:

- A patient reporting metamorphopsia around the fixation area will have difficulty eccentrically viewing. This patient will need light, high contrast, and additional magnification over the theoretical calculations made from the distant and/or near acuities.
- A patient reporting a scotoma located centrally will need further demonstrations of how to eccentrically view. This needs to be done prior to the use of optical systems.
- A scotoma to the left of, or inferior to, fixation will cause some problems in localization (getting back to the beginning of the next line). This should not preclude starting to work with a reading prescription.
- A scotoma to the right of fixation means that reading with an optical system will be difficult. The print will jump out at the patient, and localization/tracking skills will be poor. The patient needs to be taught to move the scotoma superiorly, or above the object being viewed, prior to initiating reading with an optical system. This is the best position to place the scotoma. Thus, an individual should be taught to eccentrically view superiorly (look above the reading material). Occasionally, the use of base down prism of 7^D to 10^D will make it easier for the patient to attain and sustain this optimum eccentric viewing position.

External Evaluation   This is consistent with any other external evaluation done by a primary eye care practitioner, i.e., eye movements, convergence near point, and pupil responses. These tests should be done with function in mind. Particularly if a patient is referred, function will be important, specifically to determine the use of optical and nonoptical low-vision devices. Also the type of nystagmus and presence of a null point (position of gaze where the nystagmus dampens) should be noted at this point. As with any other patient, any deviation from normal should be treated.

Internal Evaluation   This testing, although described here, is generally done at the end of the evaluation so as not to create light-dark adaptation difficulties. The extent of the internal workup will depend on the referring doctor's information, date of last internal examination, patient's report of eye changes, etc. This testing is done, not to rediagnose, but simply to confirm those pathologies that have been identified by the referring practitioner or to establish a reason for the cause of the visual impairment if self-referred. Obviously a new nonreferred patient will require a thorough evaluation for the cause of the visual dysfunction. A monocular or binocular indirect opthalmoscope with dilation is very useful for this purpose.

The referring doctor should be included as one of the team members in this vision rehabilitation process. Be careful of your statements about the pathology and about the doctor who referred the patient. If you note something of concern, depending on the severity of the problem, a letter or phone call to the referring doctor may be warranted.

Refraction   It is most important in low-vision work that the acuity losses be due to the pathology and not to an uncorrected refractive error. Thus, the next step is to perform a trial frame refraction. Cloudy media, eccentric viewing, nystagmus, reduced acuity, and poor subjective responses make the low-vision refraction more time-consuming, but not impossible. Often it will elicit different responses than the refraction performed in the primary-care setting. Neither refraction is wrong—they are just *different*!

The practitioner should take advantage of the retinoscope (radical retinoscopy at 20 or 10 cm will often help) and keratometer. Even with nystagmus, some idea of cylinder can be determined with the keratometer if the clinician remembers to move the eye to the null point and not cover the nontested eye. These objective instruments will provide a good starting point for your subjective examination. It is always best to assume the last Rx is significantly off, and/or the patient without an Rx is either a +20 diopter hyperope or a -20 diopter myope with 8 diopters of cylinder. If you establish this idea in your mind prior to the examination, you will be less likely to miss these +20D and -20D refractive errors. A more thorough discussion of the low-vision refraction is found in Mehr and Freid's *Low Vision Care*.

With the trial frame in place for the subjective refraction, use ±2.0D, ±5.0D, ±10.0D, and ±20.0D lenses with -4.0D and -8.0D cyl at each major meridian in your subjective. Stenopaic slits and pinholes are helpful tools. Remember, it may take a ±5.0D lens change to illicit a patient response. Always recheck you initial unaided or old Rx acuities to make sure the new Rx really does improve acuity. Many times the patient tries harder or has learned to eccentrically view so that the two lines with the new prescription are no better than the original prescription the patient walked in with!

Tonometry and Blood Pressure Testing   Many patients feel because they have macular degeneration or other pathologies, they are immune to other ocular problems and resist regular eye care.

Tonometry readings are necessary to make sure that intraocular pressures do not interfere with eye health and/or function. Blood pressure is equally as important to check. For in-depth information about these tests consult opthalmological or optometric texts on evaluating and treating these specific problems.

Other Tests   If other tests are needed to help give you functional information, they should be considered. Brightness acuity testing, computerized contrast sensitivity tests, electrodiagnostic testing, and interferometry, as examples, should be done if they will add to an understanding of the functional implications of the pathology.

Remember: The referring doctor will probably be following the pathology. You should concentrate on the rehabilitative aspects of the patient's care.

INITIAL LOW-VISION DEVICES EVALUATION

Once you have completed the low-vision examination, you should be ready to test your patient's ability to use various low-vision devices. The evaluation is based on the patient's particular goals. Thus, either distance or near low-vision devices should be evaluated. Ultimately, both distance and near might be evaluated, but the patient's goal should be addressed initially. Not all individuals may be able to reach their goals. Keep in mind the availability of other rehabilitative sources as well as other nonvisual means of communication, i.e., talking books, radio, etc.

You should start with magnification derived from either the distance acuity, near acuity, or a combination of the two. Remember that these acuities may be modified by information from Amsler Grid testing, lighting conditions, and any other factor you think might make a difference in the patient's success.

The sequence you develop will be personal. Remember, though, to move toward the patient's goal.

Distance Low-Vision Device Evaluation

Patients with 20/100 acuity or better should be presented with a 2.5x monocular telescope. A patient's acuity would be expected to improve 2.5 times, i.e., 20/100 VA (visual acuity) should increase to approximately 20/40. Patients with acuities between 20/100 and 20/300 should be shown a 4x or 6x unit, and those with acuities from 20/300 to 20/600 should be shown an 8x unit. Persons with acuities worse than 20/600 should not be considered for telescopes. They may be candidates for binoculars and/or special training.

VA	Telescope
20/100 or less	2.5x
20/150 - 20/300	4x–6x
20/300 - 20/600	8x–10x
20/600 or more	none

To help your patient at distance you should focus the telescope on the material first and then present it to the patient. Have the patient find you and then follow you to the chart. This will reduce the patient's initial frustration in trying to locate a small chart in a big room through the small field afforded by the telescope. (*Note*: Nystagmus is not a contraindication to successful use of telescopes. A white ring painted on the ocular housing will improve fixation.) The best responses are indicated when the patient obtains the appropriate increase in acuity and has minimal difficulty in locating objects through the device. Persons who respond well but cannot localize or focus with the device may need long-term training. Telescopes can easily be dispensed with appropriate training to the patient who demonstrates in this initial evaluation an ability to use the unit.

Utilizing the telescope in this diagnostic sequence will provide you with information on the response of the patient to telescopic magnification, to the use and appearance of the telescope, and the potential for using a telescope to solve the patients' specific problems.

Near Low-Vision Device Evaluation

As indicated earlier, evaluation of the initial near acuities can be performed utilizing the Lighthouse Near Acuity Test. There are also other charts which can be used. You will eventually settle on a chart with which you are comfortable. However, for this discussion we will continue to use the Lighthouse chart. This chart records acuities in M-notation and is designed to aid you in selecting the appropriate level of magnification. It has large isolated letters and will promote success for the initial measurement.

The patient should hold the card at a distance of 40 cm and read the smallest line possible. For the initial diagnostic sequence, the endpoint acuity of 1M (20/50) is arbitrarily selected. Since M notations are linear, if the patient reads 5M print and 1M is desired, 5x magnification is required. The print is moved to 1/5 distance or 8 cm (i.e., 40/5 = 8 cm) to obtain this magnification. A +12.5D lens is needed to provide a clear image at this distance (available accommodation may allow a weaker spectacle lens in the final Rx). This lens represents 5x magnification. To simplify the process, the chart indicates the dioptic power of the lens needed to provide 1M acuity. Thus, for the patient reading 5M, the notation is +12D in the right-hand column of the chart. This is the lens that should be placed in the trial frame. The patient is instructed to read the chart at the appropriate 8.5 cm working distance. (The card should be presented at 8.5 cm, and the patient then moves it in and out slowly to see if a better focus is obtained.) Deviations from the appropriate working distance may be indicative of uncorrected distant refractive errors, accommodation, etc. For instance, if the patient reports clear vision at 6 cm instead of 8 cm, this would indicate a possibility of 4.5 diopters of uncorrected myopia. The 6 cm indicates a demand of 16.6D (100/6 = 16.6D) instead of 12D. The difference could be 4.6 diopters of uncorrected myopia.

If the patient cannot respond to any letters at 40 cm, hold the chart at 20 cm and then use twice the indicated dioptic value from your microscopic trial lens. The use of trial lenses and a microscopic trial kit will allow you to demonstrate microscopic magnification from +4 to +100 diopters (Volk, Designs for Vision, Coburn, etc.)

A demonstration of improved acuity should be accomplished with almost every patient you see. Additionally to help others understand the functional use of the magnifier you should refer to the Freeman Functional Near Field Chart (form 2.5). This clearly demonstrates the small field of view that accompanies the improvement in acuity.

Once the level of magnification is determined utilizing the Lighthouse chart, a second acuity measurement of reading ability should be taken. A patient who can see 1M single letters may or may not be able to read equivalent size paragraph material. There are many reading cards available. Use the one you are comfortable with and hold it at the same working distance as with the Lighthouse chart. Start the patient reading a paragraph twice as large as the letters read on the Lighthouse chart. Poor performance on the reading card may

1. indicate a need for more magnification,
2. demonstrate a need for eccentric viewing training,
3. show a resistance to the close working distance, or
4. simply present an academic problem with the reading task (as in the patient who has not read in 10 years).

THE LIGHTHOUSE NEAR ACUITY TEST

DESIGNED WITH SLOAN LETTERS FOR
TESTING SUBNORMAL VISION AT 40 CM 16 INCHES

DIOPTERS OF ADD FOR AVERAGE PRINT
(1M, J #5, 9 Pt.)

DISTANT EQUIVALENT

PRINT SIZE IN METERS	ACUITY AT 40 CM IN CM	Letters		Distant Equivalent	Diopters
16M	40/1600	R K	C S	5/200	40D
13M	40/1300	Z H	D O	5/160	32D
12M	40/1200	D K	H N	10/300	28D
10M	40/1000	D S	V N	10/250	24D
8M	40/800	R H	Z C	10/200 — 20/400	20D
6M	40/600	K O	N H	20/300	16D
5M	40/500	H N O	R C V	20/250	12D
4M	40/400	C Z H	S D K	20/200	10D
3M	40/300	V R N H Z	D C S K O	20/150	8D
2.5M	40/250	H N O R C	Z S V D K	20/125	6D
2M	40/200	N R C Z H	O V S D K	20/100	5D
1.6M	40/160	D H Z V K	R C O S N	20/80	4D
1.2M	40/120	R N H S O	K D C Z V	20/60	3D
1M	40/100	V R N H Z	D C K S O	20/50	2.5D
.8M	40/80	S O C Z N	H R V D K	20/40	2D
.5M	40/50	O O S R N	S R H Z N	20/25	1D

Near vision is tested at 40 cm with best distance correction. If accommodation is insufficient add +2.50.

For visions less than 5/200, test at 20 cm and add +5.00.

"Diopters of add" are an approximation based on reciprocal of visual acuity.

LHNV-1

THE LIGHTHOUSE LOW VISION SERVICE   111 E. 59th St. NEW YORK, N.Y. 10022

Reproduced courtesy of The Lighthouse Low Vision Service.

Filter Evaluation

Evaluating filter systems must be individual. The patient may be able to give you a feel for what is comfortable in the office and even outside of the office during your initial evaluation, but for a true evaluation the patient should be allowed to borrow the filters for a few days. This allows the patient to experience the filters in everyday environment. When the patient returns, you will then know whether the filters are appropriate or need to be darker, lighter, or a different shade. Noir, Corning, and Younger are the most commonly used filters for evaluation. Remember to consider the factors of glare control, light transmission, and wavelength (color) when deciding on a specific filter.

Conclusion

At this juncture the patient is encouraged to think about what has transpired during the evaluation. A summary of the evaluation and findings are given and a recommendation for the patient to return for a continued evaluation and design of a training protocol, including the use of loaner equipmen,t is discussed. Form 3.7, Additional Adjustment Activities to Do While Waiting For Your First Optical Device Training Visit, is given to the patient. The patient is now better educated about low-vision services and will have a much better idea of the prognosis for success. These exercises will also keep the patient involved. At this stage a report should be sent to the referring doctor.

FORM DESCRIPTIONS

2.1 Cover Sheet

The cover sheet should be placed on the top of the patient's record before the initial examination. The cover sheet is a quick reference and summary of the patient's file and will eliminate the need to thumb through the entire record to retrieve basic information. It should be updated throughout the entire clinician-patient relationship.

2.2 Formal History

This history is a combination of the information the patient should have brought in plus a more formalized discussion of wants and needs. The information in the history should now be the starting point for the examination.

2.3 Examination Form (for Low-Vision Evaluation)

The examination form is used to help you gather information during this visit. It contains the compiled results found throughout your initial examination. This data will lead you, the clinician, through those tests necessary to establish a base for working with optical and nonoptical treatment options. At the conclusion of this examination period, the patient's prognosis for success will be established and treatment options discussed.

2.4 Low-Vision Device Evaluation

The low-vision device evaluation is used to list all devices used in testing. The device that is finally decided upon should be circled and noted for further reference.

2.5 Freeman Functional Near Field Chart

The Freeman Functional Near Field Chart was designed to demonstrate the functional size of the useable field of a near magnifier, i.e., hand-held, stand, telemicroscopic, head-borne, or electronic. The type size on the chart used should be consistent with the best visual acuities obtained with the low-vision device. The extent of the field can be demonstrated to the patient and others without having the patient read a word or grasp a concept. The chart can also be used to measure vertical fields.

This chart is not meant to plot out degrees of scotoma nor is the spacing between the numbers and letters meant to determine distance between printed letters. These charts were developed clinically by Barbara Freeman, and the distance between numbers and letters used is meant only to decrease confusion due to the crowding phenomenon. All diagnostic information should have been collected prior to this measurement.

This information is useful

1. at the conclusion of a near evaluation with low-vision devices;
2. as a teaching and training technique before prescribing a near Rx; and
3. as a method to monitor changes of a near useable field.

Instructions for Use of the Card

1. Place the card parallel to the near low-vision device and the patient's face. Make sure that the card is at the focal length of the lens. If used with a stand magnifier or closed-circuit TV (CCTV), interpose a reading or bifocal correction (when necessary) to compensate for diverging light from the stand magnifier or CCTV.
2. Position the lighting to achieve best illumination for use of the device.
3. With the patient viewing the center dot or where the center dot would appear to be, ask him/her to tell you the farthest number and letter that can be seen clearly to either side without moving the low-vision device. If there is a central or para-central scotoma, have the patient use an eccentric position to see the central area. This might produce a lopsided field but will be of value for patient awareness when performing other near tasks. This card can be used to teach eccentric viewing using conventional eccentric viewing techniques as well.
4. Measure this distance linearly on the chart, i.e., C, 3, B, 4.
5. Place a word or words in that space. The size of the letter or words should be based on the metric near point findings from

the low-vision evaluation. An alternative to placing word(s) in the space would be to take this finding and demonstrate it in a newspaper, magazine, etc. This will show the patient and others this measurement in the context of printed material. It will also show the patient how difficult hyphenated words, lengthy words, etc., will be. *It is most important to remember: seeing print size and determining a useable field is not synonymous with reading.*

6. Repeat the test vertically.

Summary   By using this card you will be able to demonstrate linear dimensions of both the horizontal and vertical useable field of the low-vision device(s) being recommended. Changing lighting, posture, vertex distance, etc., and then remeasuring the near field will help the patient to understand the importance of maintaining correct focal distances. The more the patient understands the functional/optical properties of the device, the more proficient she will become in using it.

COVER SHEET

Patient's Name_____Date_____

D.O.B. _____

Address _____

_____

_____

Medical insurance _____

_____

Co-Insurance _____

Secondary Insur. _____

Referring Doctor_____ Letter(s)_____

Diagnosis_____Code_____

Conventional Rx   OD_____

OS_____

Home Training Distance/Near

Print Size	14 pt.	1-	2-	3-	4/5-	6/7	Column
	12 pt.	1-	2-	3-	4/5	6/7	Column
	8 pt.	1-	2-	3-	4/5	6/7	Column

Near Rx   (D= Dispensed; L= Loaned)

(1)_____ Date_____ (D L)_____ Date_____ (D L)

(2)_____ Date_____ (D L)_____ Date_____ (D L)

(3)_____ Date_____ (D L)_____ Date_____ (D L)

Distance Rx

(1)_____ Date_____ (D L)_____ Date_____ (D L)

(2)_____ Date_____ (D L)_____ Date_____ (D L)

(3)_____ Date_____ (D L)_____ Date_____ (D L)

Sunfilters

(1)_____ Date_____ (D L)_____ Date_____ (D L)

(2)_____ Date_____ (D L)_____ Date_____ (D L)

(3)_____ Date_____ (D L)_____ Date_____ (D L)

Other:

2.2

FORMAL HISTORY

Concerns About Mobility/Distance Vision

Concerns About Near Vision

Visual History/Medical History/Family History

Previous Rx   Add

OD_____   _____

OS_____   _____

Illumination

Vocation/Work/Hobbies

Primary Goal

Secondary Goal

SUGGESTED PHRASING OF QUESTIONS

Mobility History

1. Do you get around alone outdoors, even in unfamiliar places?
2. Do you use any mobility aids like a cane or a dog?
3. Do you have any glasses or optical aids that help you get around?
4. Do you have any difficulty getting around indoors, even in strange places?
5. Do you tend to trip over coffee tables or other low objects?
6. Do you tend to bump your head on objects above your head?
7. Do you bump one side of your body more than the other?

Distance Vision History

	What Distance?	What Devise?
1. Are you able to see:		
Billboards	_____	_____
Labels	_____	_____
Faces	_____	_____
2. Do you attend movies?		
a. How close do you sit?	_____	_____
3. Do you watch TV?		
a. How close do you sit?	_____	_____
b. What is the screen size?	_____	_____
4. Do you have any problem recognizing colors?		

Near Vision

	What Distance?	What Device?
1. Do you read print?		
2. Can you read:		
a. Newspaper headlines	_____	_____
b. Large print	_____	_____
c. Textbooks	_____	_____
d. Type print	_____	_____
e. Magazines	_____	_____
f. Newspaper	_____	_____
g. Telephone book	_____	_____

3. How much reading do you do now?
4. Which type print do you use most?
5. What kind of light do you use for reading?

6. Did you read more prior to your vision loss?

7. Do you want to read more than you presently do?

Visual History

1. When did you last have an eye examination?

2. Who was your doctor?

3. Did you have treatment/surgery?

4. Are you taking eye medication?

5. Have you experienced recent changes in vision?

6. Have you ever had a low-vision examination?

7. Who was your doctor?

8. What have doctors told you caused your vision loss?

   a. Describe your problem for me.

9. How long ago did you first know you had a vision problem?

10. How well do you think you see now?

Medical History

1. When was your last physical?

2. Who is your doctor?

3. How did he/she say your health was?

4. What is your opinion of your health?

5. Are you currently taking any medications?

Family History

1. Is there any family history of glaucoma, cataract, squint, blindness, or any other vision condition?

2. Is there any family history of diabetes, hypertension, or any other medical condition?

Illumination

1. Do you see better and are your eyes more comfortable when it is bright and sunny or overcast and cloudy?

2. Do you use sunglasses?

3. Do you use a visor (hat)?

4. Are you bothered by glare?

5. Do you have more trouble with your vision at night than during the day?

6. Do you use extra light to improve your vision?

Avocation—Work/School

1. Are you involved in any of the following activities now or were you involved prior to your vision loss?

   Sewing

   Crocheting

   Playing cards

   Playing a musical instrument

   Swimming

   Bowling

   Bicycle riding

   Typing

   Computers

   Minor repairs

   Other

2. Do you have any particular difficulties at school or work because of your vision?

3. Do you have any particular difficulties around the house because of your vision?

4. How do you spend your day?

5. Tell me about some of your major activities.

6. If you improve your vision with optical devices, are there any special tasks you would like us to concentrate on enabling you to do? (Special problems?)

2.3

EXAMINATION FORM

Distance Visual Acuity (Chart:_____)

	w/old Rx	w/o Rx	Lighting
OD	_____	_____	_____
OS	_____	_____	_____
OU	_____	_____	_____

Distance Rx: OD_____ OS_____

Near Vision Acuity (Chart:_____)   (Distance_____)

	w/old Rx	w/o Rx	Lighting
OD	_____	_____	_____
OS	_____	_____	_____
OU	_____	_____	_____

Near Rx: OD_____ OS_____

Stereo Vision _____ OS_____

Color Vision: OD_____ OS_____

Binocularity_____ OS_____

Fields: OD_____ OS_____

Amsler Grid: OD_____ OS_____

EccentricViewing: OD_____ OS_____

External Evaluation   Eye movements   OD   S/J/F* Perrla Other
                                          OS   S/J/F

Keratometry   OD_____ OS _____

Internal Evaluation OD_____ OS _____

Refraction

Retinoscope   OD_____ VA_____
                     OS_____ VA_____

        Subjective   OD_____ VA_____
                     OS_____ VA_____

        Tonometry   OD_____ Test: _____
                     OS_____ Time:_____

Other Tests:

* Smooth/Jerk/Full

LOW-VISION DEVICE EVALUATION

OD	OS
Low-Vision Device(s) Distance Tested	Low-Vision Device(s) Tested
P.D.	P.D.
Low-Vision Devise(s) Near Tested	Low-Vision Device(s) Near Tested
Seg. Ht. P.D.	Seg. Ht. P.D.
Filters Tested	Filters Tested
Other	Other

16 PT. FREEMAN FUNCTIONAL NEAR FIELD CHART

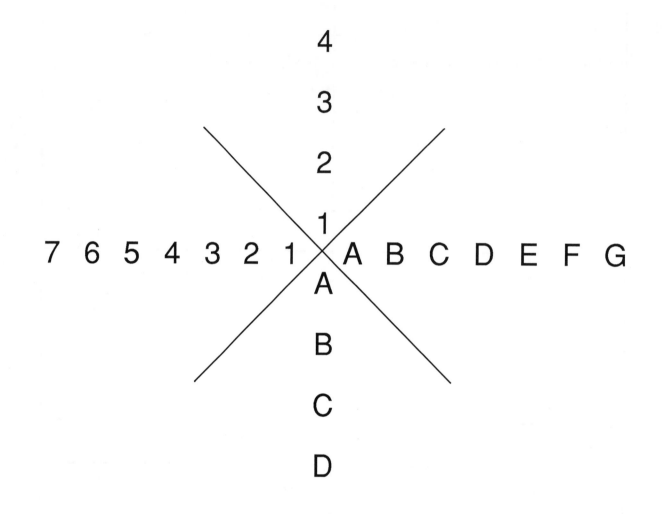

12 PT. FREEMAN FUNCTIONAL NEAR FIELD CHART

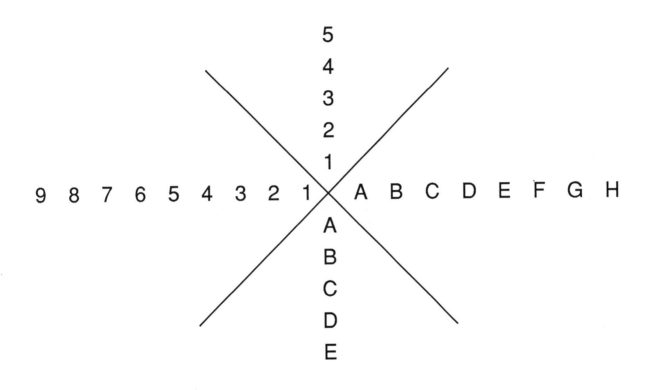

8 PT. FREEMAN FUNCTIONAL NEAR FIELD CHART

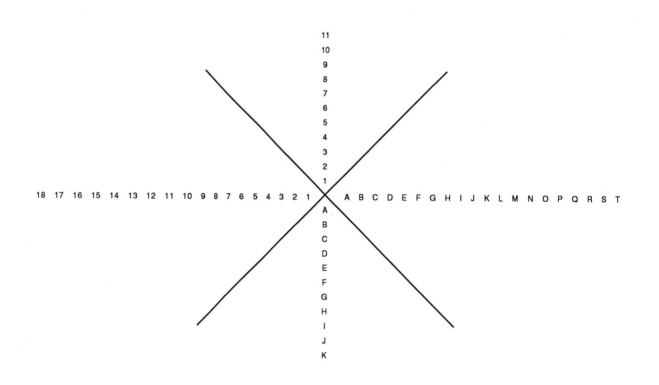

3 | After the Initial Examination

The following materials are given to your patient after the first consultation and examination. These materials recap what you should have covered in the office and give activities to span the time between visits. Even though this information is given to the patient, the individual(s) who brought the patient may have to read it to the patient. By doing so, you include significant others (spouse, parent, sibling, friend, employer) in the rehabilitation process. Two sample letters to referring physicians are also enclosed that will help you communicate the results of your examination and evaluation.

Many patients will expect to receive a pair of glasses after the first visit and may be disappointed that none were prescribed. However, as you will come to know, in most instances it is in the patient's best interest to schedule another appointment for a confirmation of findings and training. Continuing after an initial and possibly emotional first visit can cause the patient to become fatigued, reducing performance and negatively influencing success. To say this another way, "More exam can give less results." Giving the patient a break that includes activities to do at home will not only make the patient a better candidate for optical intervention but will also show your patient how active his involvement in the rehabilitation process will be. These activities should make your patient feel that something has been accomplished at the conclusion of the first visit, even if it is not obtaining the glasses as often anticipated.

CONTENTS

FORM DESCRIPTIONS

3.1 Community Services Available

This lists community resources that may provide help to your visually impaired patient. Although not an exhaustive list, this information will give you an idea of the types of services you will need to be aware of for the benefit of your patients. You will have to seek out specific agencies and organizations that provide these services in your local area and amend this list. The more active you are in the total rehabilitation process, the more your patient will benefit. You should be able to add to this list as you become more involved in low vision. It's best to have a paragraph or more about each organization and service to hand to your patient. This information should also serve as a resource to your staff.

3.2 Materials to the Patient

This is a checklist of those forms that should be given to the patient. You can add to this list as you feel the need. Note that you may need to contact some of these agencies to get the appropriate forms.

3.3 Follow-up Letter 1

A follow-up letter must be sent to the referring practitioner for two reasons. First, it helps the doctor know what has been done and how successful you were (prognosis for the patient), and it is good public relations—keeping the referral process intact. You will eventually want to develop your own style of drafting these letters, but the two examples provided here will steer you in the right direction.

3.4 Follow-up Letter 2 (See 3.3).

3.5 Your Journey Begins

The proposed examination sequence consists of three or more visits. As you know, the first visit is a consultation and diagnostic visit and is used to determine the extent of the patient's impairment. It also provides the patient with a first exposure to optical and nonoptical devices. After this visit and before you begin training the patient with low-vision systems, your patient may need a realistic pep talk. This handout will help you reinforce the concepts you discussed with your patient during the initial examination and should be given to the patient after the initial evaluation. It may have to be read to the patient.

3.6 Helping You to See Better

Some highly motivated individuals can manage, without even knowing it, to train themselves to use their remaining vision. Even as their vision becomes increasingly impaired they learn to make the best of their remaining capacity to observe critical details and shapes to help identify particular letters and numbers. They are able to pick up more information through their peripheral vision as their central vision fails. They learn to fill in letters, words, and even phrases that they can't actually see, like a detective using a few vital clues to reconstruct a crime. They also learn how to use the information they receive through their other senses to supplement the re-duced amount of information they obtain visually. More importantly, they become confident in making judgments based on these minimal cues.

But not everyone succeeds in learning these techniques on their own. The information in this handout concentrates on encouraging your patient to become aware of remaining vision and suggests techniques that can be used to stay in visual touch with the environment. These activities should be done at home between the first and second visits and are designed not only to help the patient become more visually efficient but also to keep the patient actively involved in her own rehabilitation. *Note that these activities, as most of the others, are for patients with central sight losses.*

3.7 Additional Activities to Do While You Are Waiting for Your Next Visit
This handout should also be given to the patient (along with Your Journey Begins and Helping You to See Better) after the initial consultation and diagnostic visit. It contains a series of home exercises to be used without optical devices and will introduce your patients to motor tracking skills at close working distances (specific to head-borne devices) and techniques for using telescopes at a distance. The handout gives the patient contin-ued contact with your office between the initial visit and the next visit, when you will loan the patient optical prescriptions to help begin active vision rehabilitation.

3.8 Certificate of Legal Blindness
This form documents legal blindness. This is proof of entitlement to certain benefits.

3.1

COMMUNITY SERVICES AVAILABLE

Blindness and Visual Services (Vocational Rehabilitation)

Home Health Care, Inc.

Health Department

Visiting Nurses Association

Senior Health Program

Community Health Nursing Services

Alcoholics Anonymous

Departments of Social Services

Department of Health and Human Services

Family Service Center

Family Outreach Centers

Psychiatric Hospital

Child Guidance Center

Transportation

Meals on Wheels

Sheltering Arms

National Association for the Visually Handicapped

Library of Congress

Senior Citizens Taxi Program

Head Injury Foundation

Taping for the Blind

Handicap Parking Information

Voting Assistance Hotline

Educational Services Centers

National Association for Parents of Visually Handicapped Children

MATERIALS TO THE PATIENT

Information	Date Given to Patient
Certification of Legal Blindness	
Amsler Grid	
American Diabetes Association Membership	
Radio Information Services	
Large Print Materials	
Telephone (Free Information)	
Outreach	
Macular Degeneration Association	
Retinitis Pigmentosa Association	
Transportation Services	
Talking Books	
Catalogue for Nonoptical Aids	
National Organization for Persons with Albinism and Hypopigmentation (NOAH)	
Council for Citizens with Low Vision	
National Association for Parents of Visually Impaired (NAPVI)	

3.3

FOLLOW-UP LETTER 1

(Date)

Dr. John Doe
00 Fifth Avenue
Keystone Fifth Bldg.
Pittsburgh, PA 15213

Dear Dr. Doe:

Thank you for referring Jane Smith for a low-vision consultation. I evaluated her on January 2, 1991.

My test results indicate the following:

Snellen visual acuities at distance with present lens prescription: OD 20/200, OS 20/200,
OU 20/100

Metric visual acuities at 40 cm with present lens prescription: OD 4M, OS 4M

Confrontation fields at 1M: OD full, OS full

Amsler Grid Testing at 13 inches: OD normal, OS superior left blur

External evaluation: Eye movements full but hesitant in all quadrants; Pupils responsive to light.

Lighting conditions for testing distance and near: 100 foot candles (or hi - med - low)

Internal evaluation: Consistent with macular degenerative changes

Standard refractive findings: presently conventional lenses will not alter distance or near visual
acuities.

Tonometry: OD 16, OS 16   Test:_____   Time:_____

Telescopic refraction: With a 2.2x full diameter telescope, _____ was able to
see 20/50 letter by letter with both the right eye and left eye.

Low-vision aid evaluation: Near; with a 4x (40 cm standard) microscope, was able to see 1M
print with the right eye and 1M print at 4 inches with the left eye.

Filter evaluation: Presently filters are not indicated.

Impressions and Recommendations:

Based on my findings and Jane's desires to do close activities, I am going to begin a vision rehabilitation program for her using full diameter microscopes.

Thank you very much for referring this interesting patient. Stay well.

Sincerely,

Note: Sometimes all these tests are not necessary.

FOLLOW-UP LETTER 2

Date:_____

_____

_____

_____

RE:_____

Dear Dr. _____ :

Per your referral, your patient, _____, was seen at the Low-Vision Center for a consultation visit on _____. As you know, _____ is visually impaired due to _____. Our intake indicates this impairment has created a handicap for_____ in the following areas

    1.

    2.

    3.

These were the issues addressed at this consultation visit. Today's examination indicated the distant acuities to be

    OD _____

    OS _____

    Chart used: _____

At near, the best corrected acuity is_____ in the better (right/left) eye. Color vision is (abnormal/within normal limits) as tested by large disc D-15. Contrast sensitivity screening indicates that contrast (will/will not) be a significant limitation to the successful use of low-vision prescriptions. Binocular vision tests show this patient to be (monocular; binocular; biocular) at distance and (monocular; binocular; biocular) at near. The response to optical intervention was (excellent/good/poor) at (distance/near/distance and near). Specifically,_____.

Based on today's evaluation, I am convinced that_____ will have a (poor/guarded/good/excellent) prognosis for optical intervention and vision rehabilitation services. Appropriate (appointments/follow-up contacts) will be initiated by my office. I will keep you informed of all our interactions with your patient.

I appreciate your referral of_____ to the Low-Vision Center and thank you for allowing me the opportunity to share in your patient's vision care. If I can answer any additional questions regarding _____, please feel free to call me at the office.

Sincerely yours,

3.5

YOUR JOURNEY BEGINS

The easy segment of your journey to discover useful remaining vision has been completed. Through this initial comprehensive low-vision evaluation, you and I were able to determine that you have useful sight and that optically we can maximize the use of that sight. However, now the hard part of the journey is about to begin.

Why will this part be hard? You are going into unfamiliar territory. Anytime we go from familiar to unfamiliar we have nothing to refer to or guide us. Not only is it hard but it can, and usually does, produce some anxiety. This anxiety can cause frustration. At times you may be angry or depressed. These feelings and thoughts are normal, because they are your way of coping with the work you are about to engage in. Also, as you travel this journey, you may decide to quit, but now at least you know you have options and alternatives for seeing. The phrase, **nothing can be done to help you improve your sight** is obviously wrong. You will have to decide, as you travel along this new path, whether or not you stand to gain anything so that the energy and time you spend will be worth your while. Obviously if you feel the time and energy is not going to be productive for you, you should stop.

While you are unique, others have been in similar *visual* circumstances—each having made the decision whether or not to continue. Most, however, end up feeling better for having gone this far and most develop personally satisfying "new ways of seeing."

You are the one who can make this choice. You are in charge.

Guarantees

What are your guarantees on this journey? There are no guarantees or promises except that you will be putting in time to do those things that you want to accomplish visually. To decide what you want, you will have to set goals. Take the time right now to list your goals. During the course of your training, however short or long that may be, you will always see the relevance of what you are doing. While I cannot guarantee success, I as a low-vision specialist, have worked with people like you and have helped them to achieve their journey's goals through knowledge of the pathology and functional implications of the eye condition that has created this visual problem. My staff and I will also help you set new goals as we work together.

Structuring Your Goals

Your goals may require you to be flexible. The adjustments you make will be based on many factors, but some obvious ones will be your philosophy of life, your values, and your beliefs. Remember to try to keep your goals reasonable and recognize that on your journey small steps are going to be significant to your ultimate goal. Also, remember if you don't see the relevance, it's time to stop and change directions or stop and choose alternative methods of reaching your goals.

It is important during this time, and anytime, that you feel in control of what you are doing—that you are in fact the master of your visual destiny. You are the coordinator, and the outcome of the journey you are about to begin is dependent upon your motivation, desires, and goals.

What's In It For Me?

Only you know how you feel. Your personality is unique not only because of your eyes but because each and every one of us is different. I've mentioned over and over again that the work you will be doing is tough, and it will be. When you accomplish tasks with your low-vision device—feel proud. Realize that it isn't necessary to embrace this new method of seeing, but that to accomplish your goals you will have to make changes. Also remember that you are still a person with all the traits you had before this difficulty with your visual system occurred, and you'll be that person for the rest of your life. Hopefully, what you do visually will enhance all the good qualities that make you the person you are.

Support From Others

Coping with a visual difficulty can be made easier through support from family, friends, doctors and any other people who are significant in your life. *Support does not mean "doing for you,"* but rather understanding what your difficulties are and being available when necessary. Remember those who support you will be there when you need them. They, just like you, should maintain life as usual so that undue stress is not created for anyone. Try to remember that your life was balanced among different activities before your visual difficulty. Now you should try to achieve that balance again.

Even with support, it is important for you to be an advocate for yourself. Don't be afraid to speak up—be assertive, not aggressive, when it comes to letting people know what things will make life easier for you. If you do, it will help make it easier for others to communicate with you. Keep in mind that your visual impairment doesn't make you any less intelligent, just possibly more reliant on others for some activities.

A Final Note

The work we share in getting you back on the path to usable vision is a speciality. That's why you were referred here. Once we are done, you will still need routine and continued care for your eyes. If you have other medical problems, those need to be monitored as well. Therefore, it is important that you maintain a relationship with all your regular doctors; internist, ophthalmologist, optometrist, etc.

Finally, as far as your eyes are concerned, no one can be sure how long your eyes will remain stable. Some people experience a vision loss and then stabilize for the rest of their lives, while others may experience a series of vision losses over time. Therefore, it is important to monitor your vision and, if you notice a change, your family eye doctor should be consulted. When you have been told that those services have gone as far as possible, then a phone call to us is appropriate. We will always be here when you need us.

Good Luck!

HELPING YOU TO SEE BETTER

This information is designed to help you view around blind spots or areas of decreased vision. These suggestions should help make things a little easier for you in your everyday experiences.

Scanning

If you've ever seen a celebrity at a party, or a powerful executive at a business meeting, you've seen the technique of scanning in action. Elizabeth Taylor would never walk into a room and focus her eyes solely on the person who happened to be standing in front of her. Instead, she would dart glances in all directions, checking to see who else was there, who they were with, and whether they had noticed her entrance. Good drivers also use the technique of scanning. Rather than looking only at the road directly ahead, they look off to the sides, checking for a car that might emerge from a driveway, a parked car that might suddenly swing open a door, and the way traffic is moving at the next stoplight.

Scanning is a dynamic technique. People with vision loss can use it to pick up information that they can't obtain by looking directly at people or things. They see best by looking out of the corners of their eyes, and the continual eye movement of scanning helps them to do this. This type of scanning can only be done if side vision is still available to be used.

Eccentric Viewing

The static version of scanning is to view an object by looking out of the corner of the eye. This is called eccentric viewing. A pitcher who appears to be looking directly at home plate but really is watching the runner at first base out of the corner of his eye is practicing eccentric viewing. So is the teacher who looks at the blackboard while checking on two students passing notes in the back of the classroom.

Practice: Learning to view eccentrically is a little more difficult than learning to scan, so it's a good idea to practice while you're sitting in a familiar room. Try to look at an object right in front of you: a vase of flowers, a picture, or the face of a friend. It will probably appear blurry, or even invisible, erased by the blank spot in your central vision. Move your eyes to the left or right, up and down, until you find the angle that gives you the clearest picture. You might also try moving the object closer to your eyes, or farther away, to initially establish the best distance for viewing.

Once you have learned the best angle and the best distance, you can use them to locate other objects in the room. At first, eccentric viewing will seem strange to you, but with practice, that angle will start to feel easier and more natural. You will find that you are seeing much more than you thought possible.

Practice: After you know this angle, practice using it so that you consistently use it. Now combine this with scanning. Here are two activities that may help:

1. Slowly roll a brightly colored tennis ball back and forth with someone. Use your eccentric vision to track it as it comes to you and goes away from you. This also helps with eye-hand coordination.
2. You can even practice while sitting in a restaurant or a shopping mall. Pick out a person walking by and use your eccentric viewing angle so that you see the person's head as clearly as possible and then visually follow that person. Practice will help you learn to do things easier and faster.

Practice: The next step is to practice eccentric viewing while you are moving around. It's best to begin in a familiar environment where the lighting is good. It may be very difficult at first because we humans have a strong tendency to walk in the direction our heads and eyes are pointing. So initially you'll probably veer off to one side or the other rather than walking in a straight line. Just remember that your old way of walking was learned over years of repetition, so it may take a while to learn this. But practice will pay off and you'll soon be walking confidently at the same time you are using eccentric viewing to see all around you.

Practice: Using eccentric viewing also calls for relearning your old habits of eye-hand coordination. At first you will find it hard to reach for something when you are looking at it out of the corner of your eye. Practice with an unbreakable object on a nearby table. Sight the object with eccentric viewing and then reach for it. Noticeable improvement should come in only a few practice sessions.

What you are really learning as you practice is a new relationship to your environment. Instead of confronting things directly where your central vision can offer very little help, you approach your environment from a different angle, using scanning and eccentric viewing. Your side vision will provide the visual information you need.

Eventually, you will learn the exact size and location of the blank spots in your vision. Then all you need to do is shift that blank spot away from the area you want to see. It is best if you can move the blank spot above or below the object you want to see.

Some Other Suggestions

- Learn to read body language as a substitute for facial expressions. Perhaps you can no longer make out the minute changes in expression around another person's mouth or eyes, but you can still detect such tell-tale body movements like an impatiently tapping foot, crossed arms that signal a lack of openness to the subject being discussed, or a posture that leans toward the speaker and thus indicates agreement.
- Try writing without looking at the paper. Your hands have learned the habit of writing, and they will probably continue to write legibly if you concentrate on remembering how to write rather than on trying to see what you are writing. Visualize the words in you mind's eye. For guidance in keeping the lines straight, you can buy paper with raised lines that you can feel with your hand or paper with heavy black lines you may be able to see.

A final note on these activities—**practice**. You will have to unlearn habits of seeing that you have spent a lifetime forming: the way you look at the pavement when you walk, the way you hold the newspaper to read, the way you turn your head to look at something that catches your interest. You began learning these patterns as an infant and then reinforced them with a lifetime of practice. Expect that it will take **at least** a few months of real work to teach yourself new habits.

ADDITIONAL ACTIVITIES TO DO
WHILE YOU ARE WAITING FOR YOUR NEXT VISIT

Because the lenses we usually choose to use are unconventional, they are probably going to require

1. learning to readjust the distance from your eyes to the activities you wish to do, and
2. learning to view through a smaller field than you are used to.

Between now and your next visit you may want to try a few activities at home that will acquaint you with some of the adaptations you are going to make with the lenses you will be using.

For Near

1. Every time you think of reading, writing, sewing or any close activity bring both hands to approximately_____ inches from your face. Get your muscles used to remembering this distance and forgetting the 13 to 16 inches that you've previously used for doing your close work. The more you teach your muscles these memory skills, the easier it is going to be to use your lenses for close work.
2. When you have your hands at the approximate distance noted above, move both your hands simultaneously from side to side. Imagine that you are reading, sewing, etc. You will no longer be moving your head or simply your eyes. Your eyes will remain stationary and your hands will move the imaginary page in front of you.

Over time you will learn techniques that will be suitable for you. These basic techniques will enable you to begin to understand the distance and method of being able to look at an object, and the ability to scan it at close range.

For Distance

1. When thinking about looking in the distance, curl your fingers as if looking through a spy glass. Then put that hand up to your better eye with this simulated hand telescope and look through it. Then move your head around with this new telescope and try to locate objects. This will get you acquainted with the opening and visual field you will be looking through for distance seeing.

2. Get a tube from a paper towel roll and repeat the same procedure as in #1. In addition, try to follow moving objects with this simulated telescope.

3.8

CERTIFICATE OF LEGAL BLINDNESS

I hereby certify that I have examined _____ on _____/_____/_____
and know (him/her) to be blind within the meaning of the definition set forth below.

Definition of blindness: The term "legally blind" means an individual whose (1) central visual acuity does not exceed 20/200 in the better eye with correcting lenses, or (2) that the widest diameter of the visual field subtends an angle no greater than 20 degrees.

(Code section 25 (b) (1) (c) of the Revenue Act of 1948)

_____

Signature   Date

4 | The Second Visit

During the second visit, acuities can be reevaluated and verified, more in-depth visual field testing can be performed, and refraction can be repeated, especially when a patient has diabetes, is a child, or has multiple handicaps. Any test results that were questionable can be repeated. However, the majority of time should be used to determine a tentative optical device that will begin to address the patient's previously identified needs. This chapter includes the materials you will need to effectively prescribe a low-vision device. The devices described are categorized into microscopes, magnifiers, telemicroscopes, telescopes, and electro-optical systems. This information should help you understand the functional characteristics of these systems rather than prompt you to try to memorize the thousands of devices available. It will also help you decide which device to try after another has been rejected.

In-office training with an optical system should start on the second visit to ensure that the patient understands the use of the apparatus and can appreciate both the real benefits and limitations of using the device.

When you are comfortable with your patient's ability, home training exercises should be given (see Chapter 5). You will need a loaner device from your inventory and training materials (provided in Chapter 5) to give the patient. Additional visits will be necessary until the patient demonstrates competence with the loaner. A final prescription can then be discussed based on the success of the training and goals achieved. Remember, even if a patient has more than one goal, address only one goal at a time to avoid confusion.

TREATMENT OPTIONS AND PRESCRIBING RATIONALE

When the examination has been completed, you, the clinician, must be able to utilize this data to determine an appropriate low-vision prescription. Typically at the second examination or visit

- the case history will reveal those tasks most important to the patient, i.e., goals;
- the acuity has determined the level of magnification required to see the detail necessary to perform those tasks;

- visual fields will indicate the presence of any scotomas that will make it difficult for the patient to perform those tasks;
- binocular testing will indicate the need for a monocular or binocular correction; and
- contrast sensitivity will indicate the need for special high-contrast materials and even suggest the design of better light-collecting optical systems such as full-field microscopes instead of half-eyes, etc.

The factors below are the functional optical characteristics that the clinician must consider at the second visit when deciding which of the hundreds of devices available is most appropriate for the patient. They can be summarized as:

- Magnification
- Field of view
- Lighting
- Work distance
- Mobility

Every optical system has its own advantages and limitations. These must be appreciated relative to the functional considerations listed above. The properties for all devices on the market can be summarized by dividing all optical systems into five categories:

1. Telescopes
2. Microscopes
3. Magnifiers
4. Telemicroscopes
5. Electro-optical systems

In addition there are a number of nonoptical devices that complement the optical prescriptions by

- providing greater comfort (reading stands, etc.)
- enhancing contrast (filter paper, typoscope)
- reducing glare (sun Rx, visors)

You should contact all the distributors listed in the Appendix and make yourself familiar with as many of these types of devices as possible. Remember a 100-watt light bulb can be as instrumental to successful reading as a $3000 closed-circuit television.

Telescopes

- hand-held telescopes
- clip-on telescopes
- spectacle telescope—bioptic
- spectacle telescope—behind the lens
- spectacle telescope—full field
- binoculars

Optical System Advantages and Limitations

Device	Magnification needed	Field of view needed	Work distance required	Mobility required
Microscope (MS)	Practical in +8 to +48 diopter. Special doublets preferred +32 to +80 diopters.	The full field microscope provides the largest field of view for comparable magnification. Half-eye or bifocal design will result in some loss of field of view, but will allow for mobility.	Has the shortest work distance of any system for comparable magnification.	Full-field design precludes mobility. Half-eyes or bifocals allow mobility but reduce field of view advantage.
Magnifier (MG)	2x to 5x is practical as hand magnifier. Above 5x (+20), use stand magnifier or pocket magnifier.	The magnifier is a compromise between the large field of the microscope and the small field of the telemicroscope. The patient can adjust the work distance/field of view to suit personal comfort.	Magnifiers allow a more normalized work distance and acceptable field of view for comparable magnification. This advantage dissipates at 8x magnification and above.	Magnifiers are portable and do not interfere with mobility. Acceptable for use in public.
Telemicroscope (TSMS)	Practical only up to 8x magnification (32D). Can design as a binocular with cap for greater power.	Provides the smallest field of view of all devices for comparable magnification.	Has the longest work distance for comparable magnification. Usually not a practical field of view, 6x and above, with surgicals and/or bioptic design.	Full-field precludes mobility. Surgical design allows for travel and mobility, but severely reduces field.
Telescope (TS)	Hand-held systems practical up to 10x. Bioptic design practical up to 6x. Above 10x, consider binoculars (monocular).	Not applicable; all are used for distance. A focusable telescope suffers a loss of field of view over the use of caps when used as a near telescope.	As a distance device, a telescope has a small field of view. A bioptic will have the smallest field of the types of telescopes typically prescribed. Hand-held systems provide a larger field of view. Consider binoculars (monocular). Fields 6 degrees and less are typically not practical. Keplarian telescopes have a larger field of view than Galilean.	Full-field precludes mobility, especially above 2x. Bioptic design, while reducing field of view, allows for travel, mobility, and even driving.
Electro-optical	System is practical from 8x to 60x.	For higher magnification, it allows a more normalized work distance. May need reading correction with CCTV.	The words moving across the screen give the patient an apparent larger field of view as it allows for faster information processing.	The system precludes mobility. Materials must be brought to the system for magnification. There are some portable systems, but to date, they are not very successful.

- contact lens telescope
- IOL (intraocular lens) telescope

Telescopes are prescribed for distance tasks or those tasks that have a work distance of 10 feet or greater.

Of the devices on the market, they will have the smallest field of view for comparable levels of magnification. As a starting point, you should assume the need for 20/40 distant vision. If the best corrected acuity is 20/200, then the telescopic magnification needed is 200/40 = 5x. You will find that telescopes are typically available in 4x or 6x. (You can, however, get a 5x from Designs for Vision.) It is usually best to start with the lower power (4x) as it will be easier to use the scope because of field size. This will encourage success. Remember, with a 4x the acuity will only improve from 20/200 to 20/50 (200/4 = 50). If the 6x is used next, you can expect an acuity of approximately 20/30 (200/6 = 33). For beginning any training or taking an acuity, it is best if you initially focus the telescope on the chart or object. Remember the field of view is small, and motion parallax (speed smear) is confusing to the novice patient.

Functionally, a hand-held telescope will provide an adequate field of view up to 10x (10 x 30). You should remember that the shorter the vertex distance (the closer the scope is held to the eye), the greater the field of view. Typically, a telescopic field less than 6° is not very practical for most patients. Also the greater the power, the less the field of view. Manufacturers compensate for this law of optics by making the telescopes physically larger. Thus, you can expect an 8x hand-held telescope to be a substantially larger system than a 4x hand-held system. Also, because the telescope is hand-held, mobility is no problem. Hanging it around the neck can make it more convenient to use for mobility. One limitation of a hand-held system is that it requires one hand to be occupied during use. Also it is not convenient if it has to be taken out of a pocket or purse to be used. This inconvenience obviously makes it less likely that it will be used regularly during the day. If the task required both hands to be free, a bioptic telescope can be prescribed. This is a miniaturized telescope mounted (usually) in the upper portion of a spectacle carrier lens. While this type of telescope allows both hands to be free, it severely reduces the field of view due to its miniaturized form. Remember it is produced small for placement in the carrier lens of a regular frame. If, however, a larger field is needed, this option can be made in a larger-diameter telescope and can be mounted in the carrier lens as a full-field system. This allows the proper magnification, work distance, and field of view but now prevents the person from being mobile. The patient can't look around the telescope for normal travel, and it is not efficient if the person needs to be mobile. To satisfy the needs of magnification, large field, and mobility, a clip is placed on a hand-held telescope so that it can be attached to a conventional prescription. All parameters can be met—correct magnification, work distance, and field of view. Mobility is allowed by removing the clip or by flipping the telescope up and out of the way when walking around using the regular glasses. Clipping the telescope to the glasses allows both hands to be free in addition to providing a larger field of view than a comparable bioptic system. The larger lenses also collect more light and are beneficial to those patients with contrast sensitivity problems and/or eccentric fixation problems. Drawbacks are 1. a longer vertex distance, which will make a smaller field of view than if the same telescope were hand-held, and 2. fragile stability of the system.

If after all these considerations a larger field of view is needed, binoculars should be considered. These are physically bigger and so will have a larger field of view and better light-gathering capabilities. If both hands need to be free or the patient tires easily holding these, a tripod or lap pole can be used to hold the binoculars more comfortably for extended periods.

In summary, a rule of thumb to follow is hand-held telescopes are adequate up to approximately 10x, bioptics up to approximately 6x and binoculars up to approximately 18x. This will give you a wide range of magnification options for distant tasks.

The previous discussion about manipulating the parameters of a telescope is the first phase of developing a treatment plan for your patient's distant needs. You can see that with a reasonable working knowledge of devices, you can effectively prescribe the appropriate system. Comparing these systems for similar tasks will also help you to have a better understanding of the functional optical parameters.

Two other types of telescopes are the contact lens telescope (high minus contact lens with an aphakic spectacle Rx at approximately 20 mm vertex distance) and the IOL telescope. These systems allow limited magnification up to 2x but enjoy a large field of view. The contact lens telescope requires the patient to move about with constant 2x magnification (and spatial distortions). The newer IOL systems will allow both telescopic viewing and pseudo-phakic viewing. The IOL system is still experimental and must be managed by the surgeon and low-vision clinician team. The Appendix includes references for further information on this special prescriptive technique.

Microscopes

- single-vision or doublet full field
- executive or Ben Franklin bifocal
- round seg bifocal
- Fresnel bifocal
- half-eyes
- myopic near correction
- contact lenses
- Ary Loupe

Microscopes are used for those tasks that will allow for close work distances of 2 to 20 cm. They provide the largest field of view of all systems for comparable magnification, especially when prescribed as a single-vision or doublet microscope. The field is reduced in the bifocal form of a microscopic correction, but the bifocal design allows for some mobility. (One cannot walk around wearing a +20D full-field microscope). Obviously the larger executive style or Ben Franklin style bifocal will provide a better field of view but will still make mobility more difficult. A 22-mm round seg will make it easier to walk around but may make it very difficult to localize through the microscope because of the small field of view. If the patient is in a sedentary job at a desk, the Ben Franklin would probably be the choice. If the patient is in a stock room and occasionally needs to see an invoice, the 22 round seg would be the choice. A compromise is the half-eye. It gives a larger field of view, and by sliding the lenses down the nose also increases the magnification. There are other choices if the patient can tolerate the decrease in contrast; a Fresnel lens can be used to design a large field bifocal very inexpensively. Also a monocular contact lens providing +20D of add is possible. This gives a very large field of view and allows the patient to use eye movements to read (which are very limited behind a +20 spectacle lens). However, unless the patient is biocular and can use the other eye for distant and other tasks, this is not a practical application. Another interesting system is a reverse half-eye, used for highly myopic patients. It allows the patient to look under the myopic correction and enjoy a natural magnification (a -16.00D myope enjoys 4x magnification at approximately 6 cm work distance). Using the myope's own refractive error as a near prescription provides maximum contrast (no lenses to lose light). Another way to work with a myopic patient is as follows. Correct a 20 diopter myope with a -12.00 contact lens, leaving a +8 add for reading. For distance, a -8 spectacle prescription can be designed for this patient.

Remember, the decision on which microscopic magnification system should be prescribed should be considered in view of the magnification needs, field of view, and work distant requirements as well as the importance of mobility to the task.

As a note, binocular corrections in microscopes are generally practical up to +12.0D. Prism is usually included (base in) with a standard half eye. A full-diameter system will also need a prism and will be very heavy.

Finally, if a larger field of view than a bifocal is needed and mobility is required, a Loupe/A is the choice. It clips to the distant glasses and provides a full-field system. For mobility, the patient flips it up and walks around with the distant correction. Sometimes the simpler the device, the better!

Let's again review magnification factors. Microscopic power is usually denoted in the D/4 system using 25 cm as the relative standard distance. This means a +20 diopter lens provides 5x (20/4 = 5x). However, some of the new European devices use the formula D/4 + 1 which means +20 lens is a 6x (20/4 = 5 + 1 = 6x). It's best if the clinician works with diopters to eliminate all confusion. If a patient sees 5M at 40 cm, then 1M will theoretically be seen at one-fifth that distance (40/5 = 8 cm) or 8 cm. At 8 cm a +12.5 diopter add is needed for clear vision. (In this scenario, the +12.5 lens is a 5x microscope). If the patient sees 5M at 25 cm with a conventional prescription, then 1M will be seen at (25/5 = 5 cm) 5 cm. This requires a +20D add and 5x in this system is a +20D lens. This little exercise should make it clear why it is easier to work in diopters and centimeter work distances.

Magnifiers

- hand-held
- stand
- illuminated
- mirror magnifier
- bar magnifier

Magnifiers are used as a compromise between the longer working distance of a telemicroscope and the field of view of a microscope. Their disadvantage is that they do not allow hands-free utilization. Keep in mind that with magnifiers the longer the working distance, the smaller the field of view. The patient will usually find a compromise working distance that he is comfortable with and that provides a reasonable field of view. Mobility is not a problem, since magnifiers are not attached to spectacles. Also, these magnifiers are portable.

Magnification is available in stand magnifiers and hand-held magnifiers up to dioptric value of approximately +20D. Some of the stand system are illuminated. If lighting or contrast problems exist, halogen lighting is extremely valuable. Above +20 diopters, the lens design is either a pocket magnifier or a high-power stand magnifier. Both have a very small field of view and require the patient to hold the material very close to the eye. Remember, when working with stand magnifiers, the power written on the box is usually more than the effective power of the system when used by the patient. Also keep in mind, the aphake or older patient must use a bifocal to obtain optimum magnification from most stand magnifiers (3.0 to 4.0 diopters). This is in contrast to a hand magnifier which is held at the focal length of the system and should be viewed through the distance part of the patient's prescription. There are exceptions and you must check with the manufacturer. As an example there are stand magnifiers (Coburn Blue Line) that require the patient to use the distant correction for optimum magnification.

It is interesting to note that many patients will initially prefer using a magnifier to obtain the longest work distance. However, with use they usually find that as they bring it closer to the eye, the field gets larger and they can read faster. Eventually they use the magnifier at the spectacle plane. They come back to you wanting the power of the magnifier in a pair of glasses. You can give them the microscope they turned down initially because of the short work distance. Magnifiers are often used as secondary prescriptions to complement microscopes. The microscopes are used for long-term tasks and the magnifier for more public, short-term tasks.

Telemicroscopes

- reading or surgical telescope
- bioptic telemicroscope
- clip-on telemicroscope
- hand-held telemicroscope
- binocular telemicroscope

Telemicroscopes are used for tasks requiring intermediate work distances of 20 to 100 cm. The telemicroscopic design is essentially a distant telescope modified for near use by focusing for near or by the addition of a plus cap on the objective lens. The focal distance of the plus cap dictates the work distance (+4 cap = a work distance of 25 cm). The total power of the telemicroscopic system is the power of the telescope times the power of the cap. In the 25 cm relative standard distance magnification formula, a +8 cap equals 2x magnification (D/4 = 8/4 = 2x). If we use a 4x telescope and add a +6 cap (6/4 = 1.5x), the work distance is 16.6 cm and the total magnification is 6x (4 x 1.5x = 6x). A comparable microscope would be 24D (4 x 6 = 24D) as every 4 diopters equals one times magnification in the D/4 or 25 cm relative standard distance system. A +24 lens will have a work distance of 4 cm (100/24 = 4.16 cm). Thus the telemicroscope will provide an increased work distance from 4 to 16.5 cm and still maintain the 6x magnification required for the task. The disadvantage is the severe loss of field of view. The task and patient's visual skills in compensating for the small field will dictate its usefulness as a prescription.

The telemicroscope can be designed as a full-field spectacle or clip-on telemicroscope to try to improve the field of view. The larger the telescope, the larger the field of view. To that end, placing a cap on one side of a pair of binoculars and mounting it on a tripod for stability will provide a reasonable field of view and still maintain the needed magnification. For some tasks requiring a large field of view, this is practical, for others it is not.

Electro-optical

- Closed circuit television systems

The closed circuit television system (CCTV) is a unique device that needs some special attention as a prescription. It combines relative size and relative distance magnification features, requires either a reading lens or accommodation, and needs to be manipulated using an XY table. This system provides an excellent field of view for doing close activities and maintains high contrast. Its disadvantage is that it is typically not portable, although some newer models are making it easier to have one camera to use with several work stations. Newer models are also available that can be carried in a briefcase and, by using a hand-held scanning camera, project information on a small 4 in. by 9 in. screen.

The CCTV system is a camera which focuses on reading material and transposes that material as an enlarged image to a TV screen. The patient can easily get 20x to 40x magnification and still maintain a reasonable field of view and enjoy a comfortable work distance. This is an important option when older people with poor motor control or those with small fields are in need of high levels of magnification (8x or more). The reading material moves across the screen, and the patient does not have to eccentrically view or track to process information. It's very effective, but caution should be used in using it with younger children or students as it does inhibit learning some visual skills and can make it difficult for them to adapt to the more practical hand-held systems.

Additional Prescribing Considerations

In addition to the considerations just discussed, the clinician must also give attention to some secondary factors when prescribing:

1. appearance of the system
2. cost factors
3. need for a refractive error correction
4. availability of the device
5. stability of the disease entity

After all the other factors have been worked out and you've found the perfect solution, one of the above factors will create havoc. Many times the most perfect optical prescription will be refused by the patient because of its appearance. This usually occurs with telescopes. Using more fashionable frames and tints will often help. The new Coburn behind-the-lens telescope, the Designs for Vision microspirals, or the Ocutech system are examples of small systems that are relatively hidden from view. Cosmesis should become an important consideration for the clinician when determining an appropriate prescription. This factor is important for patients 8 to 80 years old.

While costs are important, you should design the optimum system for the patient, demonstrate its benefits and limitations, and then discuss costs. Let the patient make the decision about how much they want to spend, not you. *Do not look into you patient's pockets.*

If a hyperopic or myopic astigmatic correction is needed, many stock devices will not be suitable. As an example, if a high astigmatic error is present, this part of the prescription may need to be specially ordered. Also if this patient is from out of the country and is leaving, the luxury of waiting 4 to 6 weeks for an Rx is nonexistent. You may need to glue a cylindrical lens to the optical system you want to prescribe to incorporate this cylinder. Availability therefore is a strong consideration in your prescription or design consideration.

Finally there are some vision conditions which have questionable stability. As an example, a diabetic may be considered fragile from a medical perspective. This should not interfere with prescribing a device, regardless of sophistication, if the device provides optimum visual function. If the eye has been relatively stable, a prescription for improved sight should be recommended. Discuss the prognosis with the patient. For many patients, good sight with an optical system for 2 or 3 weeks is worth the financial investment. Also if a lower-powered system is introduced to the patient and there are changes, it will make it easier to adapt to a new, stronger device. It will also make the patient able to use remembered skills if total blindness is the end result.

Field Expanders

Although the majority of this book concerns individuals requiring vision enhancement, there is a population of patients with peripheral loss. These patients require a different type of enhancement. This short segmment will introduce you to available optical intervention; it is by no means exhaustive. Field enhancers should be used by only the experienced clinician and even then are generally only successful when the doctor has the support of an orientation and mobility instructor.

- loose minus lenses
- reverse-field telescopes
- prisms (Fresnel)

These systems are designed to enhance field awareness, not to revitalize lost field. They are difficult to work with as powers needed are usually found by trial and error and clinical judgement. They require extensive practice the patient, especially to reestablish environmental relationships.

A minus lens is typically used as a hand-held system positioned away from and in front of the user. The minus lens minifies and compacts the environment so that more information is placed within the patient's constricted field. By seeing more, although minified, mobility can become safer.

Reverse field telescopes are similar to minus lenses and can be either hand-held or mounted in glasses. The telescope minifies the world placing information within the patient's constricted field. Placement of these systems should be out of central vision but useable with minimal eye movement.

Prisms can be used with either sector-field losses or constricted fields. They work by bending light, thus making information accessible to the useable portion of the retina. Typically, the prism is placed on the carrier lens over the field-loss side only, with the apex toward the center of the lens, and positioned away from straight-ahead vision. This eliminates diplopia when the patient is in primary gaze. Placement should be convenient to minimal eye movement for successful use. References related to proper placement of prism, as well as minus, lenses and reverse- field telescopes are included in the Appendix.

This is an overview of a prescribing rationale that will allow you to determine an appropriate device for your patient and evaluate that device in terms of the requirements of the task and the functional properties of the optical system. Further experience in prescribing will come with additional patients, consulting with your colleagues, and reading. The Appendix lists books and journals to help in this endeavor. The best advice is be patient with your patient and be creative.

Good luck!

ADDITIONAL VISITS

After the second visit, you should have a good idea about a prescription for your patient. Once the patient has demonstrated reasonable competence with a device while in the office, a loaner and home activities should be made available and the next office visit should be scheduled. The length of time between visits can vary, but 2 to 4 weeks is reasonable. When your patient demonstrates competence on a subsequent visit, her own device should be designed and ordered.

Your work is not done after your final dispensing. It is important to ascertain whether or not your services have helped the patient and whether or not the devices you dispensed are being used. Either a phone call or follow-up visit a month after dispensing is valuable. (Obviously the patient should know that you are available before that, but you will give the patient additional confidence with the work that has been done by telling her you will follow up in a month.)

Remember, the patient is also the referring doctor's patient, and your services should be consistent with a team approach, with the referring doctor as an integral part of general and routine eye care. Reports should be sent out after most visits.

5 | Low-Vision Homework Instructional Materials

This chapter contains instructions and homework handouts that you will need to give your low-vision patient at the end of the second visit (see Chapter 4 for more details on the second visit). They are used according to the patient's primary goal and should be assigned as such. Do not burden those patients capable of doing their reading or other near activities easily with these material. Remember it is not necessarily lens power that will determine this.

Be sure to explain to patients that these are training materials, vehicles to more functional activities like reading and writing. Not all your patients will be able to read conventional-size print; some may be able to read only large print. You should let the patient know what size print he is reading.

Lighting is very important to the success of your prescription. Each patient will respond differently to incandescent, fluorescent, or combination lighting. These should all be evaluated.

Finally, review the home training program instruction with the patient in the office. If possible, try to enlist the aid of someone who can give the patient feedback at home. Usually that is the same person who accompanied the patient to the office initially.

CONTENTS

FORM DESCRIPTIONS

5.1 Low-Vision Homework Instructional Materials—Near

These exercises are designed to be used specifically with loaner optical devices in a home training program. The instructions may have to be read to the patient. Remember, these activities can be used with any near system. They can also be used in the office for preliminary training and education in the use of low-vision devices. Choose the appropriate acuity size and provide materials from the simplest to the most complex. Stress correct working distances and proper lighting. In most cases, it is better to start with large print and work toward smaller print.

If steady fixation is a problem or poor eccentric viewing is noted (skips lines, poor sentence acuity versus single optotype acuity), the patient should be considered for eccentric viewing training tasks (see forms 5.1 and 5.2). Once the patient has mastered eccentric viewing, proceed to the home training instructional materials.

5.2 Eccentric Viewing I

The idea of these exercises is to make the patient, who needs the practice, conscious of eccentric viewing and proficient at maintaining an off-foveal fixation. The specific material in these exercises must be understood thoroughly by the patient in the office. Therefore, you should demonstrate the activities in the office before sending them home. Eccentric vision is difficult enough without your patient trying to figure out how to do it from the instructions alone. The instructional set on these pages may have to be read by someone other than the patient. Use patient feedback to help guide these activities. Be available by phone to answer questions. This training is difficult. This form (and forms 5.3 and 5.4) are offered in three different type sizes, 16, 12, and 8 point. A printer will understand the point notation for typesize should you want to vary the size of the print. To convert to M notation for consistency in relation to your low-vision evaluation, you can use the following conversion formula: Point size/8 = M (approximately).

5.3 Eccentric Viewing II (see form 5.2)

5.4 Low-Vision Reading Exercises

These exercises are obviously not reading training but are designed to reinforce saccadic movements by having the patient move the paper rather than the eyes. Use your judgment regarding size and complexity to determine which pages to give the patient. You can also modify the activity by including timing (i.e., with a metronome) or by having the patient circle specific letters.

5.5 Low-Vision Homework Instructional Materials—Distance

These exercise instructions are the same as those for near except they are designed for telescopes and are modified to reflect them.

5.6 Low-Vision Telescopic Exercises

The distance training materials concentrate on localization through a telescope. The patient needs to find things through a small aperture.

It's usually easier for most patients if they concentrate on one device at a time—distant or near. Make sure your patient has achieved optimum performance in the office before sending materials home.

5.1

LOW-VISION HOMEWORK INSTRUCTIONAL MATERIALS—NEAR

You have demonstrated that you are ready to work at home with home training activities. These activities are designed to help you relearn some reading skills. Reading itself is a very complex perceptual as well as visual physiological activity. It involves being able to see individual letters and words and being able to track along a line, but it also involves cognitive and perceptual skills.

These activities will start you on the road to eye tracking skills and letter, word, and number discrimination. For you to be as successful as possible, there are some hints that we would like to share with you.

1. Your home activities should be done for no longer than 15 minutes at a time. Fifteen minutes seems to be the appropriate amount of time one can initially work without becoming terribly frustrated or uncomfortable. These 15-minute work segments should be done 3 times a day, 5 days a week. As you work, if you find that 15 minutes goes by quickly and you are not having any problems, increase the number of 15-minute sessions.

2. During the 15-minute segment, make sure that the lighting is good. What we mean by good lighting is the amount of light that gives you the best acuity with the least amount of eye strain. Clinical experience has shown that lighting is very individual and what is good for one person is not necessarily good for another. It is, however, extremely important that the lighting be the best for the task you are doing.

Try using natural light as well as light from a lamp or any combination of light arrangements. Don't be afraid to move lamps in different locations, i.e., over the shoulder, directly above, or to the side. However, watch for glare—this can hinder your progress and make you uncomfortable. If you cannot correct lighting so you can do your task, let us know so that we can design a lighting system that will help make you successful. Now take a few moments to do an exercise demonstrating the importance of light.

Illumination Exercise

This activity should be done with someone who can help you appreciate lighting. As a side benefit, it may also help that person understand lighting and its effects.

Use the size and contrast reading materials sheet and experiment with the relationship of the light to the card and the card to your eyes. Start with a 60-watt bulb. If you think you need more light, you may want to increase the power of the bulb. First check to make sure the lamp will accept a stronger bulb. Sometimes, simple changes such as holding the book flat so that the full power of the light hits it can make reading possible again.

Notice in this exercise that good lighting lets you read smaller print in the top set of lines. However, if you have poorly printed material as in the bottom set of lines, lighting will not help you see the smaller print, even though it is the same size. *Using your vision requires contrast, lighting, magnification, proper use of your eyes, and most importantly, alot of patience and practice.*

3. When training, it is absolutely imperative that you do not do soin a rushed manner. You should do it when you are relaxed and happy, not tired or stressed. That way you can start your training on a positive note and leave it on a positive note. You should be dressed comfortably and your mind should be cleared of everything but the task at hand. These learning sessions are no different than any practice session to learn a new skill or perfect an old one. Just like anyone who strives to do better, your practice should be tailored with that thought in mind.

After 15 minutes of home training, you may feel tired, uncomfortable, or like your eyes are pulling. Possibly you may have a headache or your stomach may even be upset. These are all normal reactions to the initial use of any type of unconventional lens system. These feelings should lessen over time, but if they continue or worsen, it is important that you let us know.

4. The training materials you are to use while practicing with the new lenses have been given to you. The only item you need to purchase is a clipboard. Start with page 1 and see how far you can get in 15 minutes. It should get a little better each day. Don't worry if you start to memorize. When page 1 is so easy that you have no problem seeing and reading it, go on to page 2. Continue with this sequence until you are comfortable with all the training sheets. Remember, you can increase your sessions if you feel comfortable. It's best however not to do this during the first 5 days.

5. If this activity is difficult because of trying to look through a blind or blurry spot, eccentric viewing training needs to be added. Call the office and appropriate materials and exercises will be added to your present home training kit.

SIZE AND CONTRAST READING MATERIALS

The size of printed materials can greatly affect how easily

24 point

they can be read, even by people without visual problems. As you read this text

20 point

the print will get smaller and smaller. The largest print may not be as easy to read as

18 point

some of the smaller print, but the smallest print may be the most difficult to read. Reducing the

14 point

amount of light you are reading with can make reading even more difficult. Try reading this text with good reading light.

12 point

Now turn off some of the light and see if it becomes more difficult to read. You may even find that, with less light, you cannot read as far down this text as you could with better light. Good reading light is very important for everyone, but even more important for partially sighted people.

10 point

9 point

The quality of print is also very important in reading. This print

24 point

is the same size as the paragraph printed above, but the contrast has been reduced

20 point

by 50 per cent. That is, the print is not as dark, and it looks gray instead of black. You

18 point

will find that it is harder to read this print even in good lighting than it was to read the previous paragraph, and

14 point

it gets even harder as the print gets smaller. Once you read as much of this paragraph as possible, try reading it again with

12 point

some of the lights off. You'll find that you cannot read nearly as well as you could with better lighting. Good lighting and good reading materials are very helpful to everyone, but may be the difference between reading and not reading for the partially sighted person.

10 point

9 point

6. Visualizing what you want to do is a great way to help you to learn to do an activity better. During the course of the day you may want to practice visualizing what it will be like to successfully hold materials for reading, sewing, playing cards, viewing distance objects through a telescope, etc. Following these simple instructions will help you to visualize your activity. You may want to visualize 1 to 2 times a day. Here are the steps (adapted from relaxation exercises done by psychologists).

1. Find a quiet, dimly lit area.
2. Sit comfortably, feet flat on the floor, arms uncrossed, eyes closed, and become aware of your breathing.
3. Start taking deep, slow breaths and say "relax" as you let each one out.
4. Concentrate on any tension in your face and around your eyes. Mentally picture this tension like a knot and then visualize this knot becoming undone and limp. You should feel your face and eye muscles relax. You may also feel your body relax.
5. Now tense these same muscles and relax them.
6. Do the same for all you muscles starting with your face and work your way down to your toes—tense first then relax.
7. Now visualize yourself in comfortable surroundings for approximately 2 to 3 minutes.
8. Mentally begin doing your training whether it's with a microscope, telescope, hand magnifier, etc.
9. Feel that you are performing the activity effortlessly.
10. When you are done mentally, put the device down and relax for approximately 30 seconds.
11. Now open your eyes and go about the rest of your day.

Work hard, but enjoy yourself.
Call if you have *any* problems or questions.

Eccentric Viewing 1
16 point with Low-Vision Device

You have demonstrated that you are almost ready to begin tracking activities that will help you with print. However, because you cannot use straight-ahead viewing, we have designed materials to help you establish the best off-center viewing spot for you.

Selecting the Best Angle for Eccentric Viewing

The following exercises will help you in selecting the best angle for eccentric viewing. Three lines of decreasing thickness are placed above each letter or word, and three lines of increasing thickness are placed below each letter or word. Starting with the single letters, select the line (above or below) the letter that allows you to see the letter most clearly. That is, you should center your vision on the line that gives the clearest view of the letter in your peripheral visual field. The following few pages of training materials provide lines of the same height to help you learn eccentric viewing.

E

An

16 pt.

Remember to use your best angle of vision for reading the following materials. Scan each word slowly saying it aloud. It is more important to use your best viewing angle than it is to read fast. Your reading speed will improve later as you get used to reading this way.

are   key   way

may   the   its

any   see   who

16 pt.

5.2a continued

This page is a little more difficult because the words are longer and closer together. Remember, accuracy in using your best viewing angle and in reading each word correctly is still more important than how fast you read.

were	then	seen	ride

list	have	mean	word

with	loud	care	make

fair	open	band	race

16 pt.

This is the last training page. Learning to use your vision is not easy, but it will become easier and you will enjoy reading more.

white   green   black   brown   color

phone   crumb   paste   paint   burnt

while   family   ready   meant   makes

carry   dealt   carve   gravy   great

16 pt.

Eccentric Viewing 1
12 point with Low-Vision Device

You have demonstrated that you are almost ready to begin tracking activities that will help you with print. However, because you cannot use straight-ahead viewing, we have designed materials to help you establish the best off-center viewing spot for you.

Selecting the Best Angle for Eccentric Viewing

The following exercises will help you in selecting the best angle for eccentric viewing. Three lines of decreasing thickness are placed above each letter or word, and three lines of increasing thickness are placed below each letter or word. Starting with the single letters, select the line (above or below) the letter that allows you to see the letter most clearly. That is, you should center your vision on the line that gives the clearest view of the letter in your peripheral visual field. The following few pages of training materials provide lines of the same height to help you learn eccentric viewing.

E

An

12 pt.

Remember to use your best angle of vision for reading the following materials. Scan each word slowly saying it aloud. It is more important to use your best viewing angle than it is to read fast. Your reading speed will improve later as you get used to reading this way.

are	key	way
may	the	its
any	see	who

12 pt.

This page is a little more difficult because the words are longer and closer together. Remember, accuracy in using your best viewing angle and in reading each word correctly is still more important than how fast you read.

were	then	seen	ride
list	have	mean	word
with	loud	care	make
fair	open	band	race

12 pt.

This is the last training page. Learning to use your vision is not easy, but it will become easier and you will enjoy reading more.

white	green	black	brown	color

phone	crumb	paste	paint	burnt

while	family	ready	meant	makes

carry	dealt	carve	gravy	great

12 pt.

Eccentric Viewing 1
8 point with Low-Vision Device

You have demonstrated that you are almost ready to begin tracking activities that will help you with print. However, because you cannot use straight-ahead viewing, we have designed materials to help you establish the best off-center viewing spot for you.

Selecting the Best Angle for Eccentric Viewing
The following exercises will help you in selecting the best angle for eccentric viewing. Three lines of decreasing thickness are placed above each letter or word, and three lines of increasing thickness are placed below each letter or word. Starting with the single letters, select the line (above or below) the letter that allows you to see the letter most clearly. That is, you should center your vision on the line that gives the clearest view of the letter in your peripheral visual field. The following few pages of training materials provide lines of the same height to help you learn eccentric viewing.

E

An

8 pt.

Remember to use your best angle of vision for reading the following materials. Scan each word slowly saying it aloud. It is more important to use your best viewing angle than it is to read fast. Your reading speed will improve later as you get used to reading this way.

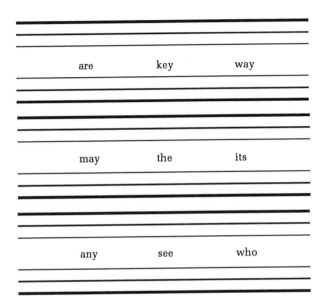

8 pt.

5.2c continued

This page is a little more difficult because the words are longer and closer together. Remember, accuracy in using your best viewing angle and in reading each word correctly is still more important than how fast you read.

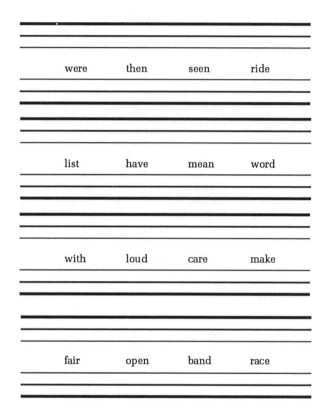

were	then	seen	ride
list	have	mean	word
with	loud	care	make
fair	open	band	race

8 pt.

This is the last training page. Learning to use your vision is not easy, but it will become easier and you will enjoy reading more.

| white | green | black | brown | color |

| phone | crumb | paste | paint | burnt |

| while | family | ready | meant | makes |

| carry | dealt | carve | gravy | great |

8 pt.

Eccentric Viewing II
16 Point with Low-Vision Device

You have demonstrated that you are almost ready to begin tracking activities that will help you with print. However, because you cannot use straight-ahead viewing, we have designed materials to help you establish the best off-center viewing spot for you.

This is designed to help you determine an oblique angle of fixation. The materials have the following form:

━━━━━━━━

─────

────

123456789

────

─────

━━━━━━━━

16 pt.

The horizontal angle for fixation is determined in the same way as the previous section. The oblique angles use the diagonal created by the edges of the three horizontal lines. The top lines are for those fixating above objects, and the bottom lines for those fixating below objects. The edges on the left can be used for those fixating behind the object to be viewed, while the edges on the right can be used for those fixating ahead of an object. For reading tasks it is best to try to move the blind spot superiorly. These fixational skills may be important for activities other than reading.

Selecting the Best Angle
for Oblique Eccentric Viewing

The following exercise will help you determine the best angle of viewing. Three lines of decreasing thickness are placed above each group of numbers or letters and three lines of increasing thickness are placed below them. Starting with the first group of numbers, select the line above or below the numbers that best allows you to see the numbers. The diagonal edges (top left and right, and below left and right) can be used to determine the best oblique angle. For example, using the middle line below the number centers your eyes on the left edge of the line. What numbers can be seen? Center on the right edge. What numbers can be seen now? One position will usually be better than the other and this is the angle you should practice using. The letters and combinations of letters and numbers on this and subsequent pages can be used to confirm the angle and/or serve as additional practice materials.

1234567   ABCDEF   1A2B3C4

16 pt.

The following exercises are designed to help you improve your reading capability. Use the reference lines that worked best for you on the previous page. Concentrate on using your vision as accurately as possible and don't worry yet about your reading speed. Increased speed will be gained with training materials that follow this one. Right now, it is more important to be accurate than fast.

when   zoom   must   bang

seed   even   boot   time

must   fair   cold   heat

16 pt.

Eccentric Viewing II
12 Point with Low-Vision Device

You have demonstrated that you are almost ready to begin tracking activities that will help you with print. However, because you cannot use straight-ahead viewing, we have designed materials to help you establish the best off-center viewing spot for you.

This is designed to help you determine an oblique angle of fixation. The materials have the following form:

```
━━━━━━━━
 ───────
   ─────
123456789
   ─────
 ───────
━━━━━━━━
```

12 pt.

The horizontal angle for fixation is determined in the same way as the previous section. The oblique angles use the diagonal created by the edges of the three horizontal lines. The top lines are for those fixating above objects, and the bottom lines for those fixating below objects. The edges on the left can be used for those fixating behind the object to be viewed, while the edges on the right can be used for those fixating ahead of an object. For reading tasks it is best to try to move the blind spot superiorly. These fixational skills may be important for activities other than reading.

Keep Practicing

Selecting the Best Angle
for Oblique Eccentric Viewing

The following exercise will help you determine the best angle of viewing. Three lines of decreasing thickness are placed above each group of numbers or letters and three lines of increasing thickness are placed below them. Starting with the first group of numbers, select the line above or below the numbers that best allows you to see the numbers. The diagonal edges (top left and right, and below left and right) can be used to determine the best oblique angle. For example, using the middle line below the number centers your eyes on the left edge of the line. What numbers can be seen? Center on the right edge. What numbers can be seen now? One position will usually be better than the other, and this is the angle you should practice using. The letters and combinations of letters and numbers on this and subsequent pages can be used to confirm the angle and/or serve as additional practice materials.

1234567   ABCDEF   1A2B3C4

12 pt.

The following exercises are designed to help you improve your reading capability. Use the reference lines that worked best for you on the previous page. Concentrate on using your vision as accurately as possible and don't worry yet about your reading speed. Increased speed will be gained with training materials that follow this one. Right now, it is more important to be accurate than fast.

when	zoom	must	bang

seed	even	boot	time

must	fair	cold	heat

12 pt.

Eccentric Viewing II
8 Point with Low-Vision Device

You have demonstrated that you are almost ready to begin tracking activities that will help you with print. However, because you cannot use straight-ahead viewing, we have designed materials to help you establish the best off-center viewing spot for you.

This is designed to help you determine an oblique angle of fixation. The materials have the following form:

123456789

8 pt.

The horizontal angle for fixation is determined in the same way as the previous section. The oblique angles use the diagonal created by the edges of the three horizontal lines. The top lines are for those fixating above objects, and the bottom lines for those fixating below objects. The edges on the left can be used for those fixating behind the object to be viewed, while the edges on the right can be used for those fixating ahead of an object. For reading tasks it is best to try to move the blind spot superiorly. These fixational skills may be important for activities other than reading.

Keep Practicing

Selecting the Best Angle
for Oblique Eccentric Viewing

The following exercise will help you determine the best angle of viewing. Three lines of decreasing thickness are placed above each group of numbers or letters and three lines of increasing thickness are placed below them. Starting with the first group of numbers, select the line above or below the numbers that best allows you to see the numbers. The diagonal edges (top left and right, and below left and right) can be used to determine the best oblique angle. For example, using the middle line below the number centers your eyes on the left edge of the line. What numbers can be seen? Center on the right edge. What numbers can be seen now? One position will usually be better than the other and this is the angle you should practice using. The letters and combinations of letters and numbers on this and subsequent pages can be used to confirm the angle and/or serve as additional practice materials.

1234567   ABCDEF   1A2B3C4

8 pt.

The following exercises are designed to help you improve your reading capability. Use the reference lines that worked best for you on the previous page. Concentrate on using your vision as accurately as possible and don't worry yet about your reading speed. Increased speed will be gained with training materials that follow this one. Right now, it is more important to be accurate than fast.

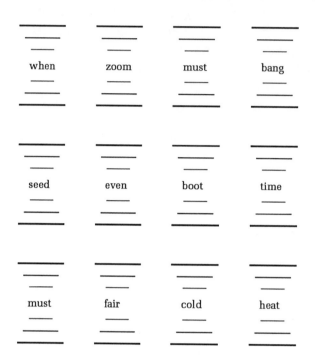

when	zoom	must	bang
seed	even	boot	time
must	fair	cold	heat

8 pt.

LOW–VISION
READING EXERCISE—16 pt.

W S I M J Z D L T V T D Z M S G I R L X

J Z W O N Q B F S L G X R E F B P H Z F

T P K J S W Z N I W K U T D S B R E E B

P H K N D W Q T Z P J A Y H B M I R A Q

S V T D M T K Z Y V W K W A Y G X M Z Q

i g s o w y u n k v q t b p l e r d n z o m w

f k u j r j g x i q z v l p t d n z o m w p b z

r w u c m e j g x q i z v l d e b v p t q l e d

r x e m r u y k n q b t p q d r x h z f g i s o

w e x s l u j k l d x z m j i s w y n k q u o g

g q o c x l f e r y a j p n q m k l t r s o p e t

w e s l t x m w z z j m q n o w c i m k t l n

x r j f i c w a y h b f s u c m m i r a x c m z

m e w j w r z n t b t p u o h g a j y p h b c o

g q o j k y s x d x z b n y u g w a e s b x t l

LOW–VISION
READING EXERCISE—16 PT.

up it in he me on is be no or do go on we

he we am or in we it an if as do of in so

no go on do of or is to we he up it or me

up so go we at am in we he on of so if as

me we is as it am if an we go do up or at

or do up is as he in am at of up go if is

in of up as if an it me in or am we he is

or it up he we on is or to do go on no we

no go do or no be is on as he it in up or

or up do go we an if am it we is he me if

of go no or an do it is me up he or go me

up he go or on is we if he it or do go me

to we as if an in he me am is up or do go

of go up or to am in he as we is me go at

is of do as if an it me in or am we he in

LOW–VISION
READING EXERCISE—16 pt.

yes its not let too may saw run men off who

our add red ago had air the any was all yet

and his way got try set six how she has old

out did put top car sea can too use boy you

but dog why end say eat sun for own few far

not run off man say may too try its who yes

yet all was any the air set let got way his

old has she ago six had get red how add our

can you why boy car say sea new cut did out

far few own for sun eat top end use dog but

got way his try six set had she how her has

now red ask any air set the ago men was are

him who its too let man say all not run off

but dog top man sun few yes eat far own end

men not run may saw let day too him who yes

LOW–VISION
READING EXERCISE—16 pt.

well stand want would went ready work house

peace well which show right much green hear

ever under will point such group same happy

until eyes paper when given most south made

said parts even going were north some table

place hand great each clear what thing high

more order head wrong done trees with often

found away train home today door front very

sure horse less times help night days never

woman real those live early here earth does

used funny room might life eery have apple

think true means read close land three grow

call miles told could page comes left their

money cold black turn young play there last

give being town years took shown part lives

LOW–VISION
READING EXERCISE—16 pt.

animals another within united against

because between making brought places

during country children behind certain

different bigger example writing friend

following second plants however himself

inside important learned cannot looking

across morning saying nothing letters

school picture though perhaps heating

remember letter started several family

something sentences became almost sometimes

through thought turned sentence person

others usually living without together

baseball change working program better

reading wetter states herself brother

newspaper beautiful really outside number

LOW–VISION
READING EXERCISE—16 pt.

a	make
and	me
away	my
big	not
blue	one
can	play
come	red
down	run
find	said
for	see
funny	the
go	three
help	to
here	two
I	up
in	we
is	where
it	yellow
jump	you
little	
look	

LOW–VISION
READING EXERCISE—16 pt.

all	out
am	please
are	pretty
at	ran
ate	ride
be	saw
black	say
brown	she
but	so
came	soon
did	that
do	there
eat	they
four	this
get	too
good	under
have	want
he	was
into	well
like	went
must	what
new	white
no	who
now	will
on	with
our	yes

LOW–VISION
READING EXERCISE—16 pt.

about	laugh
better	light
bring	long
carry	much
clean	myself
cut	never
done	only
draw	own
drink	pick
eight	seven
fall	shall
far	show
full	six
got	small
grow	start
hold	ten
hot	today
hurt	together
if	try
keep	warm
kind	

LOW–VISION
READING EXERCISE—16 pt.

always	or
around	pull
because	read
been	right
before	sing
best	sit
both	sleep
buy	tell
call	their
cold	these
does	those
don't	upon
fast	us
first	use
five	very
found	wash
gave	which
goes	why
green	wish
its	work
made	would
many	write
off	your

LOW–VISION
READING EXERCISE—16 pt.

from home

I will go

the little children

will look

you are

all night

her father

the red apple

in the garden

what I say

the little chickens

will think

you were

all day

her mother

the red cow

about him

as he said

did not fall

LOW–VISION
READING EXERCISE—16 pt.

the yellow ball	to the school	can live
has run away	will walk	it was
he was	on the chair	with us
up there	so long	has made
your mother	the new doll	the black bird
a big horse	could make	by the house
to the house	he would do	if you can
he would try	when you come	can run
the old man	to the barn	from the tree
went away	was made	they are
we are	in the box	at once
down here	to go	will buy
his sister	the funny rabbit	the small boat
some cake	a big house	in the barn
from the farm	when I wish	as I said
as he did	you will like	can fly
the old men	in the grass	to the farm
was found	must be	they were
we were	in the window	at three
up here	to stop	will read
his brother	the funny man	the small boy

LOW–VISION
READING EXERCISE—12 pt.

L D X Z J M I S W Y K N U Q O G A C H F P B R E

T D Z M S N O C W I F J R X L B V E H A G U K Y

N L P K T R O W E J Q Z M C I G S E F B H A V Y

D Z T K W S Q B J F L P C Y N V E R A I M X G O

P I Z M N K T D S V U G Q C O X L F R E H B A Y

C S D T U W V K Y R G O Q N Z M I J A H F B P E

k y u w o s g i c a j m f h z r x e d l p b t v z e r t u

e l h x r a j g f u k y i s c w m o z d n q t p r z l p u

i x g j e c m t r w f o s p t b j y k a l n v d t m n o p

y l c b n j v s e k a w r i t m z q x d h g o u z m p g

s v o q d c x t k l m j z e n r i h p y j n b a w z p t

g o q y v z m w n k j u i a d h s p b c l e x m r e p

r h r f c a g o u k q n y t w s i m z j j z x d l t h v r

b y w s i j m z x d l t v p k b r e h a c o g u k f z t

v w k t d y f l b j s c l x e o g x m i r a e v n y z p

h b r f l x c o q t v b p p h a f i j r a v n y y w s g c

c s d j f k y c s m w k y r n b l h p y z r h g o r t z s

4 2 5 3 6 8 9 7 1 3 2 8 5 4 6 3 7 5 9 3 8 5 0 2 1 5

LOW–VISION
READING EXERCISE—12 pt.

so an as is do on it if we or in he am is on be up

me an is as at am to if no do it in up or we so go

do of me or so if an we if it or to no as we is he

is up or so in of do as if an it me in or am we he

is if do we is me go to an as up or at am in he as

am if an in he me as is up no to we or do go of he

an is we if he in to me up he go or or do go me in be

to of do it is me up he or go me no at go or no on

at or up do go we as is he me if no of an if am it

no on go up or he do or no be is on we he in it am

me or it up he we on is of or do go on no we it be

so in of do me in or am as if an it we he is up at

go or do up at or up go if is as he in am is do me

if me is he as it am if an we go do up or at me no

it up so go we at am in we he to of so is as or be

we of or is on we no go on do he up it or me in of

is he we if as do of am or in me it an in so go me

we so or up it in he on we is be no or do go no on

LOW–VISION
READING EXERCISE—12 pt.

far but why and yes her did add not out few new ago

put six far old air may say eat she any let sea end

its use way any dog try are him you day yes why you

who too she try saw top six use sun was sea the see

say set off old own put one now out new out add red

say far her not cut few has men air car for how ago

any can his eat had may all boy end let are big dog

its and but sea day get him can buy not you and man

put out set use sat may the let sea had its as got

him yet get one new old far own did few see cut for

car sun eat can six top and try big dog why but boy

way add now ago off air run saw any all too are who

yes run saw and its may how eat can our off too who

say own his boy use all any end put old see did boy

men how air car ago few top sun try way you one add

cut let dog way why the its six big are she red not

way day you him are dog use its all six end try not

all may had can any man how for car air eat men but

LOW–VISION
READING EXERCISE—12 pt.

ever green eyes group even given each going house

done front door found days does early first down

earth cold every city come could came black close

among book began body best below boys above both

been asked able along away wrong again also after

wind ready will right point high paper hear hard

parts head place home help often have other order

here grow might gave means give never lives good

money feel make smiles face later fire learn fish

light feet large known form kinds from hands food

your small year still half into study idea sound

story know since keep kind short knew shown space

their long these look think line three like last

those land times life today live trees thing less

most using more until make under made which many

would older went stand want place show such happy

same said wrong seen north some clear train sure

horse room woman read seven play funny page apple

LOW–VISION
READING EXERCISE—12 pt.

wetter heating baked perhaps toward picture really

nothing number morning states letters enough looking

called learned before important without himself female

however around following turned without should usually

always together living thought father through change

sentence better sometimes others something saying

bought course though started school remember people

glasses letter required family anything several outside

brother newspaper almost beautiful bigger herself friend

became wanted reading second working plants program

mother baseball inside another moving animals become

against cannot because across within between united

things brought answer children making country little

during certain behind different places example around

himself always following better however change writing

father important person learned others looking should

letters turned morning living nothing female picture

almost family became heating course remember perhaps

LOW–VISION
READING EXERCISE—12 pt.

a	make
and	me
away	my
big	not
blue	one
can	play
come	red
down	run
find	said
for	see
funny	the
go	three
help	to
here	two
I	up
in	we
is	where
it	yellow
jump	you
little	

LOW–VISION
READING EXERCISE—12 pt.

all	out
am	please
are	pretty
at	ran
ate	ride
be	saw
black	say
brown	she
but	so
came	soon
did	that
do	there
eat	they
four	this
get	too
good	under
have	want
he	was
into	well
like	went
must	what
new	white
no	who
now	will
on	with
our	yes

LOW–VISION
READING EXERCISE—12 pt.

about	laugh
better	light
bring	long
carry	much
clean	myself
cut	never
done	only
draw	own
drink	pick
eight	seven
fall	shall
far	show
full	six
got	small
grow	start
hold	ten
hot	today
hurt	together
if	try
keep	warm
kind	

LOW–VISION
READING EXERCISE—12 pt.

always	or
around	pull
because	read
been	right
before	sing
best	sit
both	sleep
buy	tell
call	their
cold	these
does	those
don't	upon
fast	us
first	use
five	very
found	wash
gave	which
goes	why
green	wish
its	work
made	would
many	write
off	your

LOW–VISION
READING EXERCISE—12 pt.

from home

I will go

the little children

will look

you are

all night

her father

the red apple

in the garden

what I say

the little chickens

will think

you were

all day

her mother

the red cow

about him

as he said

did not fall

LOW–VISION
READING EXERCISE—12 pt.

the yellow ball	to the school	can live
has run away	will walk	it was
he was	on the chair	with us
up there	so long	has made
your mother	the new doll	the black bird
a big horse	could make	by the house
to the house	he would do	if you can
he would try	when you come	can run
the old man	to the barn	from the tree
went away	was made	they are
we are	in the box	at once
down here	to go	will buy
his sister	the funny rabbit	the small boat
some cake	a big house	in the barn
from the farm	when I wish	as I said
as he did	you will like	can fly
the old men	in the grass	to the farm
was found	must be	they were
we were	in the window	at three
up here	to stop	will read
his brother	the funny man	the small boy

LOW–VISION
READING EXERCISE—8 pt.

K Q U O G C A H F P B V T D L Z X J I M S Y W N R H W S M

G S B D L X R J F C I W O N Q P T D Z V E H A G U K B Q P

W J E X Q I Z G C M S U F B H Y A V D L K N T P R O H Y I

N Y V E A R I M X G O U D H T Z K Q S W B J L F C P D O P

Q O C X F L R B E Y A W J T P N Z K M D T S V U G E R N I

A F H P B S E X F T R Q N Z M J I L M S T D L O R Z T P L E

T L D X Z J M S W N T Y R F H R P B V L E Z I U P B M N R T

a j f z h x r d a l p t b v q n k y u w s o i g m c l m s t z h l c m

c w s o m z n d t q v p b e h x l a r g i g j i r k m n p o q r t w

s p c b l e x f r g o q y n v z w k m u j i t a d h d s g l k e t y l

b s l x r f c w o n q p t d m z s y k g u a e h v k q u d p l m o n

v d t k x n v b r w i t o p w q c r u g r n l p q r s t w v y u o x n

f p u o h g d x z m e t l q r k a w e s w r c f p o z i r c r w r g l

1 9 0 2 3 4 8 5 4 7 5 8 9 1 4 3 7 6 9 4 8 3 2 5 9 7 5 6 7 2 3 4 6

1 5 u y 8 u 0 e 4 5 x 6 v 7 b 8 n 9 m 0 1 s 2 d 3 f 4 g 5 h 6 g 7 j

v d t k m z i p n j w a y h n h b r e f l x c q g u s l g i p r q w m

f p u o h g d x z m t l q r k w a s e v j n b y l f c p o z t r p u m

1 c 8 x 2 9 v 5 i b 3 r 5 o 7 p b 4 5 i v 9 j 6 m 4 r s 6 y p 3 c q

f t b p h k y n a l v d z q i x g j m e c w u r s o c k l r u b v r t y

a j f z h x r d a l w y n y r h k q u o g c a f h r p e b v z d r s l t

i 8 0 3 5 j o 8 6 j 4 p e 3 2 0 j 8 h 9 x 4 2 c v b 5 7 8 h 9 l 8 n j

9 2 8 4 7 5 0 3 1 9 6 0 3 0 6 1 7 4 8 5 3 9 2 6 8 2 4 0 1 8 8 7 4

k 5 h 6 g 0 f 8 d 4 s 1 a 2 q 5 w 0 r 3 t 5 y 7 u 5 p 7 a 3 z 8 p 0

LOW–VISION
READING EXERCISE—8 pt.

we on no go do or no is on we he in be it up or he am if

go me so in of do as is an it in or am he we is up on at

in me or it up he on is or of do we on go no we in be as

as if so of to he we in am at or we go so up it or no we

be at or up do we an if am it as is he go me if on an up

do is if go or at am in he up as is up do or go if in of

am up is he we or in me it an if as do of in so go be it

it we no go do of or is on we up it or me in as so he

he or up in it he we on is be no or do go he no on we is at

or if me he is as it am if an we go he do up or at be in

 am no me go or he up me is it do on or no go of to it we

in me go do or it he we is an or go he up me is an or if

 no to go do or up is as me he in an if am we to go is be

me is we of to go as he am at or up do if is go in on do

up is he we am or in me it an if as of in so at go to do

to or it he we as if an we is me if so or do of on be is

so we up in is an me it do no of to am or at or as he up

is am in or up be we it if on he do is at an so in go he

or at be do up we if am it an is me he go if or as me no

am up it or go so at we in he we of to if so or as be do

we on no go or do be no is on we he it in up or he at is

go no to am if an in he me as is up or we do go of in be

in so an at is do it if we up be or in he on am is on we

LOW–VISION
READING EXERCISE—8 pt.

day why dog top end for eat sun few own yes far but out

use new put did cut say sea car can you big boy our now

red get ago six had she how her has old his and got add

way set the air was any are all yet you boy use big try

sea can say car did put new out yes him who its too cut

let say man run may not off for yes far few own had saw

eat sun end top why day but off not run men may saw dog

man let too its who him yet are was all ago the set yes

air any ask red now our has her how she had six got old

try his way get and day but why end top eat sun for dog

own far few yes new out did put say car sea can use cut

boy now our add you red ago get had six how she has big

old her and his way got try set the any was all yet air

are him yes its who let too may saw run men off not man

big yes far few own for sun eat top end why dog but day

use did can you say car boy sea cut her out put old new

has she how all six try had got way his and get are yet

was any the air set ago red add run our now not off men

cut man saw may too let who its yes put him new out did

say car sea can use big boy day dog why you but and too

eat sun for own few far not off men man run may yes

yes was too set let air who the its any saw him all are yet

try way get had his six and how ago got her she old has

LOW–VISION
READING EXERCISE—8 pt.

also about from heard half must water side after wind small

your still year words away again find kinds into sound hands

more soon along able known from study idea write mean where

asked that been story food while just above name light large

they since back fast among know learn next space this world

white both below four keep short need whole them later began

boys lives five kind years near being shown then makes best

there face young knew over money time their black body comes

fish like miles only these than funny could book class feel

means think once apple take every came long might fire three

line look seven open earth tell never come those good woman

horse early part night took times city give first last order

page today turn often train cold found gave left trees play

wrong told front call other grow land clear thing read great

true north place down table have life going room parts used

south does using here live paper rest until given upon happy

days going help older point less under sure very green door

right home which many seen house with peace read done would

head stand more water small what heard each about hand said

words make were still some after where even sound high kinds

made again same write when eyes known hard along study most

while such story will ever asked hear world much since large

show light work above ways will white went space want learn

LOW–VISION
READING EXERCISE—8 pt.

making places herself things beautiful brother united

outside within moving anything across newspaper required

become glasses cannot inside started mother several remember

wanted plants sentences second something through friend

sentence bigger thought sometimes almost became together

course usually family without following letter people

school himself though important bought learned however

saying looking always change morning better letters nothing

father living perhaps others heating should another picture

animals person against turned female because around between

before brought called enough country children looked certain

different really example toward writing states number

saying heating wetter glasses moving without bigger perhaps

example required better usually within female picture

friend person different bought anything together states

newspaper noting united certain wanted though between

turned letters toward things beautiful second children

school sentence looking should brought really sometimes

places herself plants people thought others learned brother

number something important mother because making letter

reading living sentences himself little working looked

program inside several family however father against enough

LOW–VISION
READING EXERCISE—8 pt.

a	make
and	me
away	my
big	not
blue	one
can	play
come	red
down	run
find	said
for	see
funny	the
go	three
help	to
here	two
I	up
in	we
is	where
it	yellow
jump	you
little	
look	

LOW–VISION
READING EXERCISE—8 pt.

all	out
am	please
are	pretty
at	ran
ate	ride
be	saw
black	say
brown	she
but	so
came	soon
did	that
do	there
eat	they
four	this
get	too
good	under
have	want
he	was
into	well
like	went
must	what
new	white
no	who
now	will
on	with
our	yes

LOW–VISION
READING EXERCISE—8 pt.

about	laugh
better	light
bring	long
carry	much
clean	myself
cut	never
done	only
draw	own
drink	pick
eight	seven
fall	shall
far	show
full	six
got	small
grow	start
hold	ten
hot	today
hurt	together
if	try
keep	warm
kind	

LOW–VISION
READING EXERCISE—8 pt.

always	or
around	pull
because	read
been	right
before	sing
best	sit
both	sleep
buy	tell
call	their
cold	these
does	those
don't	upon
fast	us
first	use
five	very
found	wash
gave	which
goes	why
green	wish
its	work
made	would
many	write
off	your

5.4c continued

LOW–VISION
READING EXERCISE—8 pt.

from home

I will go

the little children

will look

you are

all night

her father

the red apple

in the garden

what I say

the little chickens

will think

you were

all day

her mother

the red cow

about him

as he said

did not fall

LOW–VISION
READING EXERCISE—8 pt.

the yellow ball	to the school	can live
has run away	will walk	it was
he was	on the chair	with us
up there	so long	has made
your mother	the new doll	the black bird
a big horse	could make	by the house
to the house	he would do	if you can
he would try	when you come	can run
the old man	to the barn	from the tree
went away	was made	they are
we are	in the box	at once
down here	to go	will buy
his sister	the funny rabbit	the small boat
some cake	a big house	in the barn
from the farm	when I wish	as I said
as he did	you will like	can fly
the old men	in the grass	to the farm
was found	must be	they were
we were	in the window	at three
up here	to stop	will read
his brother	the funny man	the small boy

Low-Vision Homework Instructional Materials
Distance with Low-Vision Device

You have been shown various techniques for the efficient use of telescopic systems while in the office. Now it is up to you to practice these skills at home. Before starting these activities consider these hints.

1. Your home activities should be done for no longer than 15 minutes at a time. Fifteen minutes seems to be the appropriate amount of time one can initially work without becoming terribly frustrated or uncomfortable. These 15-minute work segments should be done 3 times a day, 5 days a week. As you work, if you find that 15 minutes goes by quickly and you are not having any problems, increase your time by 5 minute segments. It is best, however, not to do this during the first 5 days. Also, it is wise not to go over 30 minutes during any one session. If you are doing 30 minute sessions comfortably, then increase the number of sessions per day. This is more productive.

2. During the 15-minute segment, make sure that the lighting is good. What we mean by good lighting is the amount of light that gives you the best acuity with the least amount of eye strain. Clinical experience has shown that lighting is very individual and what is good for one person is not necessarily good for another. It is, however, extremely important that the lighting be the best for the task you are doing. However, once you go outside, lighting will be difficult to control. Therefore, practice inside with good light until you are comfortable enough to enter an environment where you will be unable to control the lighting.

3. When training, it is absolutely imperative that you do not do so in a rushed manner. You should do it when you are relaxed and happy, not tired or stressed. That way you can start your training on a positive note and leave it on a positive note. You should be dressed comfortably and your mind should be cleared of everything but the task at hand. These learning sessions are no different than any other practice session to learn a new skill or perfect an old one. Just like anyone who strives to do better, your practice should be tailored with that thought in mind.

After 15 minutes of home training, you may feel tired, uncomfortable, or like your eyes are pulling. Possibly you may have a headache or your stomach may even be upset. These are all normal reactions to the initial use of any type of unconventional lens system. These feelings should lessen over time, but if they continue or worsen, it is important that you let us know.

4. Visualizing what you want to do is a great way to help you learn to do an activity better. During the course of the day you may want to practice visualizing what it will be like to successfully hold materials for viewing distance objects through a telescope, etc. Following these simple instructions will help you visualize your activity. You may want to visualize 1 to 2 times a day. Here are the steps (adapted from relaxation exercises done by psychologists).

1. Find a quiet, dimly lit area.
2. Sit comfortably, feet flat on the floor, arms uncrossed, eyes closed. Become aware of your breathing.
3. Start taking deep, slow breaths and say "relax" as you let each one out.
4. Concentrate on any tension in your face and around your eyes. Mentally picture this tension like a knot and then visualize this knot becoming undone and limp. You should also feel your face and eye muscles relax. You may also feel your body relax.
5. Now tense these same muscles and relax them.
6. Do the same for all your muscles starting with your face and work you way down to your toes—tense first then relax.
7. Now visualize yourself in comfortable surroundings for approximately 2 to 3 minutes.
8. Mentally begin doing your training with your telescope.
9. Feel that you are performing the activity effortlessly.
10. When you are done, mentally put the device down and relax for approximately 30 seconds.
11. Now open you eyes and go about the rest of your day.

Work hard, but enjoy yourself.
Call if you have *any* problems or questions.

Low-Vision Telescopic Exercises

Telescopic work can be extremely frustrating because unlike working at near, you do not have control over what you are viewing. So, in an effort to minimize this frustration you may want to follow this sequence of activities. Remember these are guidelines. You will find that after a while you'll develop your own strategy.

1. Locate a stationary object with your eye. Stand approximately 15 to 20 feet from that object. If you have a hand-held telescope, lift it to your eye. If you have a head-borne, lower your head while raising your eye so that you can look through the telescope.

Focus the telescope on the target. Once the target is clear, identify as much detail as you can as well as the amount of area you see. Now put the telescope down and move 5 feet closer to the target. Refocus and repeat the previous step of identifying detail and field. Continue to do this until you are as close as you can get to the target where focusing will no longer clairfy the image. Now, reverse the process.

2. Position yourself about 20 feet away from a group of separated objects to be viewed. Locate the objects first with your eye and then through the telescope. If you have a hand-held device, practice raising the telescope to your eye, viewing the targets by looking through the telescope and moving your head, then lower it. Your goal should be to move quickly and efficiently, lifting the telescope to your eye, then locating, identifying, and putting the telescope back down. If you are using a head-borne device, the same concept applies. Locate the target, look through the telescope, identify the targets, and then move your eye out of the telescope. Once you are able to do this smoothly and efficiently with either a head-borne or hand-held telescope, change distances, refocus, and repeat the procedure.

3. When stationary objects become easy to see, locate a moving target, i.e., a person or vehicle, while you are stationary. Track the target with your unaided vision, lock in on the target, and if your telescope is hand-held, lift it to your eye and track the object. With a head-borne telescope, lower your head so your eye moves into the telescope and follow the target.

4. Now that you have gotten this far, you may want to track a stationary object while moving, using the same principles.

Remember

- Once the telescope is up to your eye, objects are going to move more quickly than they would normally.
- Targets will move in a direction opposite to the movement of the telescope. If you scan to the left, the targets will move to the right and quickly. This is called movement parallax and may make you initially uncomfortable.
- Moving targets are significantly more difficult to work with than stationary targets regardless of who is doing the moving.
- If you are using a monocular system, you might initially want to close the eye that is not being used. However, over time having both eyes open will prove to be more efficient.
- In any activity you do with your telescope be sure to use the telescope in a logical and sequential scanning pattern. In the event that a target is difficult to see with the scope, first locate the area you want to view, find a stationary point around the target, bring the scope to your eye, locate that point, then sequentially scan the area until you are able to locate and identify what you wish to see.

5. Once you become very smooth at doing these activities, try to enhance your memory skills by looking through your telescope, identifying a scene, then closing your eyes and attempting to remember everything you have seen through the telescope. This will help increase your ability to get as much information as you can, as efficiently as possible.

A Last Note

The success of using a telescope depends greatly upon your motivation and how efficiently you use this device. As you use your telescope more often in your environment, your skill level will improve. Recognize that although the telescope may not be as cosmetically appealing as a designer frame, you will be performing significantly better with than without the use of this device. As in any other segment of training, if you have any problems please feel free to call us.

Good luck.

Appendix: Resources

ORGANIZATIONS

There are organizations that provide a variety of services for the visually impaired. This is only a partial list developed by the authors.

American Diabetes Association
Judith Oehler, Ph. Ed., RN
800 ADA-DISC

American Foundation for the Blind
15 West 16th Street
New York, NY 10011
(212) 620-2000
(800) 232-5463

Association of Radio Reading Services
P.O. Box 847
Lawrence, KS 66044
(913) 864-4600

Council of Citizens with Low Vision
1211 Connecticut Ave., N.W.
Suite 506
Washington, DC 20036
(202) 833-1251

Helen Keller National Center for Deaf-Blind Youths and Adults
111 Middle Neck Road
Sands Point, NY 11050
(516) 944-0900 / 944-8900
(Voice and TDD, Telecommunication Device for the Deaf)

RP Foundation Fighting Blindness (National Retinitis Pigmentosa
Foundation, Inc.)
1401 Mt. Royal Avenue
Fourth Floor
Baltimore, MD 21217
(301) 225-9409
(800) 638-2300

American Printing House for the Blind
P.O. Box 6085
1839 Frankfort Avenue
Louisville, KY 40206
(502) 895-2485

American Council of the Blind
1010 Vermont Avenue, N.W.
Suite 100
Washington, DC 20005
(202) 393-3666

Association for the Education and Rehabilitation of the Blind and
Visually Impaired
206 North Washington Street
Suite 320
Alexandria, VA 22314
(703 548-1884

Association for Macular Disease
210 E. 64th Street
New York, NY 10021

Library of Congress National Library Services for the Blind and
Physically Handicapped
1291 Taylor Street, N.W.
Washington, DC 20542
(202) 287-5100
(800) 424-9100

National Association for the Visually Handicapped
22 West 21st Street
New York, NY 10010
(212) 889-3141

National Association for Parents of Visually Impaired
2180 Linway Drive
Beloit, WI 53511
(800) 562-6265

National Organization for Albinism and Hypopigmentation
Nevil Institute for Rehabilitation
919 Walnut Street., Room 400
Philadelphia, PA 19107
(215) 627-3501

National Society to Prevent Blindness
500 East Remmington Road
Schaumburg, IL 60173
(312) 843-2020

Rehabilitation Services Administration
330 C Street, S.W.
Washington, DC 20202
(202) 732-1282

EQUIPMENT SOURCES

The practitioner may wish to write to the listed companies to initiate a list of resources and become familiar with a larger variety of optical systems available. This is a partial list as developed by the authors.

American Foundation
  for the Blind
15 West 16th Street
New York, NY 10011
(800) AFBLIND
(212) 620-2000

nonoptical low-vision devices and adaptive equipment

American Optical Company
Optical Products Division
14 Mechanic Street
Southbridge, MA 01550
(800) 225-7498
(617) 765-4711

optical low-vision devices

Bernell Corporation
750 Lincolnway East, Box 4637
South Bend, IN 46634
(800) 348-2225

optical low-vision devices

Bossert Specialties Inc.
Low Vision Aids
P.O. Box 15441
3620 E. Thomas Road, Suite d-124
Phoenix, AZ 85060
(602) 956-6637

optical and nonoptical devices and adaptive equipment

Coburn Optical Industries, Inc. P.O. Box 627 1701 South Cherokee Road Muskogee, OK 74402-0627 (800) 262-8761	optical low-vision devices CCTV, low-vision lighting systems
Corning Medical Optics Corning, NY 14831 (800) 742-5273	absorptive lenses
Designs for Vision 760 Koehler Avenue Ronkonkoma, NY 11779 (800) 345-4009	optical low-vision devices
Duffens Optical Low Vision Aids 3625 Willowbend Suite 110 Houston, TX 77054 (713) 663-3000	optical low-vision devices
Eschenbach Optik of America 25 November Trail Weston, CT 06883 (203) 227-9409	optical low-vision devices
F/V Microscopes 1500 Brodhead Road Aliquippa, PA 15001 (412) 375-7030	optical low-vision microscope
Keeler Optical Products, Inc. 456 Parkway Broomall, PA 19008 (800) 523-5620 (215) 353-4350	optical low-vision devices
Lighthouse of Houston Low Vision Aids Department 3602 West Dallas Houston, TX 77219 (713) 284-8466	writing magnifiers and specialty magnifiers

Luzerne Optical   optical low-vision systems
180 North Wilkes-Barre Blvd.
P.O. Box 998
Wilkes-Barre, PA 18703
(717) 822-3183
(800) 223-9637 (national)
(800) 432-8096 (PA)

M-Pencar Associates   lighting
137-75 Geranium Avenue
Flushing, NY 11355
(718) 939-7031

Maitland Vision Center   lighting
540 E. Horatio Street
Maitland, FL 32751
(407) 628-3133

Mattingly International   optical low-vision devices
938 K-A Andreason Drive
Escondido, CA 92029
(800) 826-4200

Mons International   nonoptical low-vision devices
Suite 200
800 Peachtree Street, NE
Atlanta, GA 30308
(404) 344-8805

NOIR   NOIR absorptive lenses
P.O. Box 159
South Lyon, MI 48178
(800) 521-9746 USA
(800) 227-3396 Canada

Ocutech Inc.   telescopes
P.O. Box 625
Chapel Hill, NC 27515
(919) 967-6460
(800) 326-6460

Optical Aid Services New York Association for the Blind (The Lighthouse) 111 East 59th Street New York, NY 10022 (212) 355-2200	optical and nonoptical low-vision devices
Optelec P.O. Box 729 Westford, MA 01886 (508) 392-0707	CCTV and low-vision reading devices
Optical Designs, Inc. 14441 Memorial Drive Suite 13 Houston, TX 77079 (713) 497-2988	optical low-vision devices
Rekindle 5462 Memorial Drive Suite 101 Stone Mountain, GA 30083 (800) 666-7484	field loss devices
Telesensory Systems, Inc. (TSI) P.O. Box 7455 Mountain View, CA 94039 (800) 227-8418 (415) 960-0960	CCTV
Walters, Inc. 30423 Canwood Street Suite 126 Agoura Hills, CA 91301 (818) 706-2202	optical low-vision devices
Younger Optics 3788 South Broadway Place Los Angeles, CA 90007 (800) 366-5367 (213) 232-2345 (Calif.)	optical low-vision devices

Bibliography

EXAMINATION

Bailey, I. L. (1978). Visual acuity measurements in low vision. *Optometric Monthly*, 69(7):418–424.

Bailey, I. L. and Lovie, J. E. (1976). New design principles for visual acuity letter charts. *American Journal of Optometry and Physiological Optics*, 53:740–745.

———(1980). The design and use of a new near vision chart. *American Journal of Optometry and Physiological Optics*, 57(6):378-387.

Baldasare, J., Watson, G. R., Whittaker, S. G., and Miller-Shaffer, H. (1986). The development and evaluation of a reading test for low vision macular loss patients. *Journal of Visual Impairment and Blindness*, 80:785-789.

Ball, G. V. (1973). Anomalies of vision in low illumination. *American Journal of Optometry*, 50(3):200-205.

Brown, B., Zadnik, K., Bailey, I. L., and Colenbrander, A. (1984). Effect of luminance, contrast, and eccentricity on visual acuity in senile macular degeneration. *American Journal of Optometry and Physiological Optics*, 61(4):265-270.

Corn, A. L. (1983). Visual function: A theoretical model for individuals with low vision. *Journal of visual Impairment and Blindness*, 77:373-377.

Cummings, R. W., Whittaker, S. G. Watson, G. R., and Budd, J. M. (1985). Scanning characters and reading with a central scotoma. *American Journal of Optometry and Physiological Optics*, 62:833-843.

Faye, E. E. (1968). A new visual acuity test for partially sighted nonreaders. *Journal of Pediatric Ophthalmology*, 5:210-212.

Ginsberg, A. P. (1984). A new contrast sensitivity vision test chart. *American Journal of Optometry and Physiological Optics*, 61(6):402-407.

Gutteridge, I. F. (1985). Clinical significance of detecting visual field loss. *American Journal of Optometry and Physiological Optics*, 62(4):275-281.

Krischer, C. C., and Meissen, R. (1983). Reading speed under real and simulated visual impairment. *Journal of Visual Impairment and Blindness*, 77:386-388.

Legge, G. E., Rubin, G. S., Pelli, D. G., and Schleski, M. M. (1985). Psychophysics of reading, II:Low vision. *Vision Research*, 25:253-266.

Loshin, D. S., and White, J. (1984). Contrast sensitivity: The visual rehabilitation of the patient with macular degeneration. *Archives of Ophthalmology*, 192(9):1303-1306.

Sheedy, J. E., Bailey, I. L., and Raasch, T. W. (1984). Visual acuity and chart luminance. *American Journal of Optometry and Physiological Optics*, 61(9):595-600.

TREATMENT OPTION

Bailey, I. (1983). Can prisms control eccentric viewing? *Optometric Monthly*, 74(7):360-362.

Bailey, I. (1982). The honey bee lens: A study of its field properties. *Optometric Monthly*, 73(5):275-278.

Bergenske, p., and Raasch, T. (1982). Bioptic low vision aid: A simple approach. *American Journal of Optometry and Physiological Optics*, 59(3):283-286.

Brown, B. (1981). Reading performance in low vision patients: Relation to contrast and contrast sensitivity. *American Journal of Optometry and Physiological Optics*, 58:218-226.

Cole, R. G. (1983). The low vision aphakic patient. *Journal of American Optometric Association*, 54(8):735-739.

Feinbloom, W. (1977). Driving with bioptic telescopic spectacles. *American Journal of Optometry and Physiological Optics*, 54(1):35-42.

Fonda, G. (1983). Bioptic telescopic spectacle is a hazard for operating a motor vehicle. *Archives of Ophthalmology*, 101(112):1907-1908.

Fraser, K., Jose, R. T., and Loshin, D. (1983). Contrast sensitivity function and low vision management: Report of a case. *Optometric Monthly*, 75(9):460-464.

Gerushat, D. (1985). Illumination and mobility. In *Orientation and mobility of low vision of individuals: A final report*. Philadelphia, Pennsylvania College of Optometry.

Goodrich, G. L., Mehr, E. B., Quillman, R. D., Shaw, H. K., and Wiley, J. K. (1977). Training and practicer effects in performance with low vision aids: A preliminary study. *American Journal of Optometry and Physiological Optics*, 54(5):312-318.

Janke, M., and Kazarian, G. (1983). *Accident record of drivers with bioptic telescopic lenses*. Sacramento, California State Department of Motor Vehicles.

Jose, R. T., Carter, K., and Carter, C. (1983). A training program for clients considering the use of bioptic telescopes for driving. *Journal of Visual Impairment and Blindness*, 77:425-428.

Kelleher, D. K. (1972). *The effect of bioptic telescopic spectacles upon the self concept and achievement of low vision students in itinerant programs*. Unpublished dissertation, University of California at Berkeley.

————(1976). Driving with low vision from the patient's perspective. *American Journal of Optometry and Physiological Optics*, 53(8):440-441.

Kleinstein, R. N. (1978). Reading with a 10x telescope. *American Journal of Optometry and Physiological Optics*, 55(10):732-734.

Levin, M., and Kelleher, D. K. (1975). Driving with a bioptic telescope: An interdisciplinary approach. *American Journal of Optometry and Physiological Optics*, 52(3):200-206.

Loshin, D. W., and Browning, R. A. (1983). Contrast sensitivity in albinotic patients. *American Journal of Optometry and Physiological Optics*, 60(3):158-166.

Lynch, D. M., and Brilliant, R. (1984). An evaluation of the Corning CPF550 Lens. *Optometric Monthly*, 36-42.

Morrissette, D. L. (1984). Large print computers: An evaluation of their features. *Journal of Visual Impairment and Blindness*, 78:428-434.

Moss, H. (1984). Red lenses and patients with rod monochromatism. *Review of Optometry*, 121:77-78.

Press, L. J. (1985). Visual perception and optical aid performance. *Journal of Vision Rehabilitation*, 1:10-12.

Romayananda, N., Wong, S. W., Elzeneiny, I. H., and Chan, G. H. (1982). Prismatic scanning method for improving visual acuity in patients with low vision. *Ophthalmology*, 89(8):937-945.

Woo, G. C., and Wessel, J. A. (1982). Use of contrast sensitivity function in prescribing low vision aids. *American Journal of Optometry and Physiological Optics*, 59(11):924-925.

TELESCOPE

Bailey, Ian (1982). The honey bee lens: A study of its field properties. *Optometric Monthly*, May, 275-278.

Berliner, Milton (1936). A new type of telescopic lens. *Archives of Ophthamalogy*, 16(4):649-654.

Biessels, W. J. (1973). Binocular low vision telescopic spectacles. *Journal of the American Optometric Association*, December, 1238-1243.

Brilliant, Richard (1984). Horizon or amophic lens. *Rehabilitative Optometry*, 2(1):14.

Browning, Robert, and Jose, Randy (1984). The low vision triangle. *Rehabilitative Optometry*, 2(1):12-14.

Byer, Alvin (1986). Magnification limitations of a contact lens telescope. *American Journal of Optometry and Physiological Optics*, 63(1):71-75.

D'Alessandro, L. (1983). Honey bee lens gives wide field of view. *Review of Optometry*, January 15, 1983, p. 74.

Feinbloom, William (1977). Driving with bioptic telescopic spectacles. *American Journal of Optometry and Physiological Optics*, 54(1):35-42.

Freeman, Paul (1980). Evaluating the needs of the low vision teenager. *Optical Journal and Review of Optometry*, 117(6):49-50.

Genensky, Samuel M. (1974). Binoculars: A long ignored aid for the partially-sighted. *American Journal of Optometry and Physiological Optics*, 51(9):648-673.

Kelleher, Dennis (1974). A pilot study to determine the effect fo the bioptic telescope on young low vision patients' attitude and achievement. *American Journal of Optometry and Physiological Optics*, 51(3):198-205.

Kelleher, Dennis (1976). A new multipurpose low vision aid. *Optometric Weekly*. August 26, 41-44.

Kestenbaum, Alfred (1962). New kinds of application of telescopic systems. *American Journal of Ophthalmology*, 53(3):443-444.

Lee, Dan, and Jose, Randy (1976). Low vision care—Not everyone wants it. *Optometric Weekly*, 67(50):1365-1369.

Levy, Alan (1980). A versatile low vision aid. *Review of Optometry*. December, 1983, p. 38.

Marks, Roy (1948). Factors concerning the prescription and use of telescopic spectacles. *American Journal of Optometry and Physiological Optics*, 25(6):262-274.

Mehr, Edwin, and Freid, Allan (1975). *Low vision care—Prescribing and counseling*, Chap. VIII. Professional Press, Chicago, IL, pp. 109-111.

Mehr, Helen, Mehr, Edwin, and Ault, Carroll (1970). Psychological aspects of low vision rehabilitation. *American Journal of Optometry and Physiological Optics*, 47(8):610-614.

Tait, Edwin, and Neill, John C. (1936). A new subnormal vision appliance. *American Journal of Optometry*, 13(2):55-60.

Walters, Gary B. (1980). A bioptic telescope clip. *Review of Optometry*, 117(8):52-54.

RESTRICTED FIELD

Bailey, Ian (1978). Prismatic treatment of field defects. *Optometric Monthly*, 60:1073-1078.

Baunschweig, P. (1922). Hemianopsia aided by prisms. *Ophthalmology Yearbook*, p. 395.

Brilliant, Richard (1984). Horizon or amorphic lens. *Rehabilitative Optometry Journal*, 2(1):14.

Drasdo, N. (1976). Visual field expanders. *American Journal of Optometry and Physiological Optics*, 53(3):464-467.

Ferraro, John, Jose, Randy, and McClain, Linda (1982). Fresnel prisms as a treatment option for retinitis pigmentosa. *Texas Optometry*, 38(5):13-17.

Finn, W. A., Gadbaw, P. O., Kevorkian, C. A., and DeL'Anne, W. R. (1975). Increased field accessibility through prismatically displaced images. *New Outlook for the Blind*, 69(10):465-467.

Goodlaw, Edward (1982). Rehabilitating a patient with bitemporal hemianopsia. *American Journal of Optometry and Physiological Optics*, 57(3):183-186.

Hoeft, W. W., Feinbloom, W., Brilliant, R., Gordon, R., Hollander, C., Newman, J., Novak, E., Rosenthal, B., and Voss, E. (1985). Amorphic lenses: A mobility aid for patients with retinitis pigmentosa. *American Journal of Optometry and Physiological Optics*, 69(2):142-148.

Holm, C. (1970). A simple method for widening restricted visual fields. *Archives of Ophthalmology*, 84:611-612.

Jose, R. (1986) (Unpublished clinical study at University of Houston College of Optometry Low Vision Clinic of 50 patients with retinitis pigmentosa.)

Jose, Randy, and Smith, Audrey (1976). Increasing peripheral field awareness with Fresnel prisms. *Optical Journal and Review of Optometry*, 113(12):33-37.

Kennedy, W., Rosten, J., Young, L., Ciuffreda, K., and Levin, M. (1977). A field expander for patients with retinitis pigmentosa: A clinical study. *American Journal of Optometry and Physiological Optics*, 54(11):744-55.

Mehr, Edwin, and Quillman, Dec. (1979). Field "expansion" by use of binocular full field reversed 1.3x telescopic spectacles: A case report. *American Journal of Optometry and Physiological Optics*, 56:446-450.

Mose, Randall, Spitzberg, Larry, and Kuether, Chris (1989). A behind the lens reversed (BTLR) telescope. *Journal of Vision Rehabilitation*, 3(2):37-46.

Neuremberg, Benjamin (1980). A new mirror design for hemianopsia. *American Journal of Optometry and Physiological Optics*, 57(3):183-186.

Rickers, K. (1978). Visual Field Wideners: A personal report. *Journal of Visual Impairment and Blindness*, 72(1):28-29.

Spitzberg, L., and Jose, R. (1988). *Fitting guide for the behind-the-lens telescope.* Optical Designs, Inc., Houston, TX.

Weiss, Norman (1972). An application of cemented prisms with severe field loss. *American Journal of Optometry and Archives of the American Academy of Optometry*, 49(3):261-264.

Weiss, Norman (1984). Adapting an automobile for a driver with hemianopsia. *Journal of Rehabilitative Optometry*, 2(3):7.

FURTHER READINGS

Faye, Eleanor (1984). *Clinical Low Vision.* Little, Brown and Co., Boston, MA.

Jose, Randy (1982). *Understanding Low Vision.* American Foundation for the Blind. New York, NY.

Kirschner, Corrine (1985). *Data on Blindness and Visual Impairment in the United States.* American Foundation for the Blind, New York, NY.

Mehr, Edwin, and Freid, Alan (1975). *Low Vision Care.* Professional Press, Chicago, IL.

Newsletter of the Low vision Section of the AOA.

The Journal of Vision Rehabilitation. Media Publications, 2440 O St., Suite 202, Lincoln, Nebraska 68510.

The Journal of Visual Impairment and Blindness. American Foundation for the Blind, 15 W. 16th St., New York, New York.

Regular articles also appear in the JAOA and JAAO.